I0114564

Culture, Politics, Ideology and Reproductive Health in Turkey

Yılmaz Esmer (ed.)

Culture, Politics, Ideology and Reproductive Health in Turkey

PETER LANG

Bibliographic Information published by the Deutsche Nationalbibliothek
The Deutsche Nationalbibliothek lists this publication in the Deutsche Nationalbibliografie; detailed bibliographic data is available online at http://dnb.d-nb.de.

Library of Congress Cataloging-in-Publication Data
A CIP catalog record for this book has been applied for at the Library of Congress.

ISBN 978-3-631-84890-6 (Print)
E-ISBN 978-3-631-87977-1 (E-PDF)
E-ISBN 978-3-631-87978-8 (E-PUB)
10.3726/b19751

Peter Lang – Berlin · Bruxelles · Istanbul · Lausanne · New York · Oxford

This publication has been peer reviewed.

www.peterlang.com

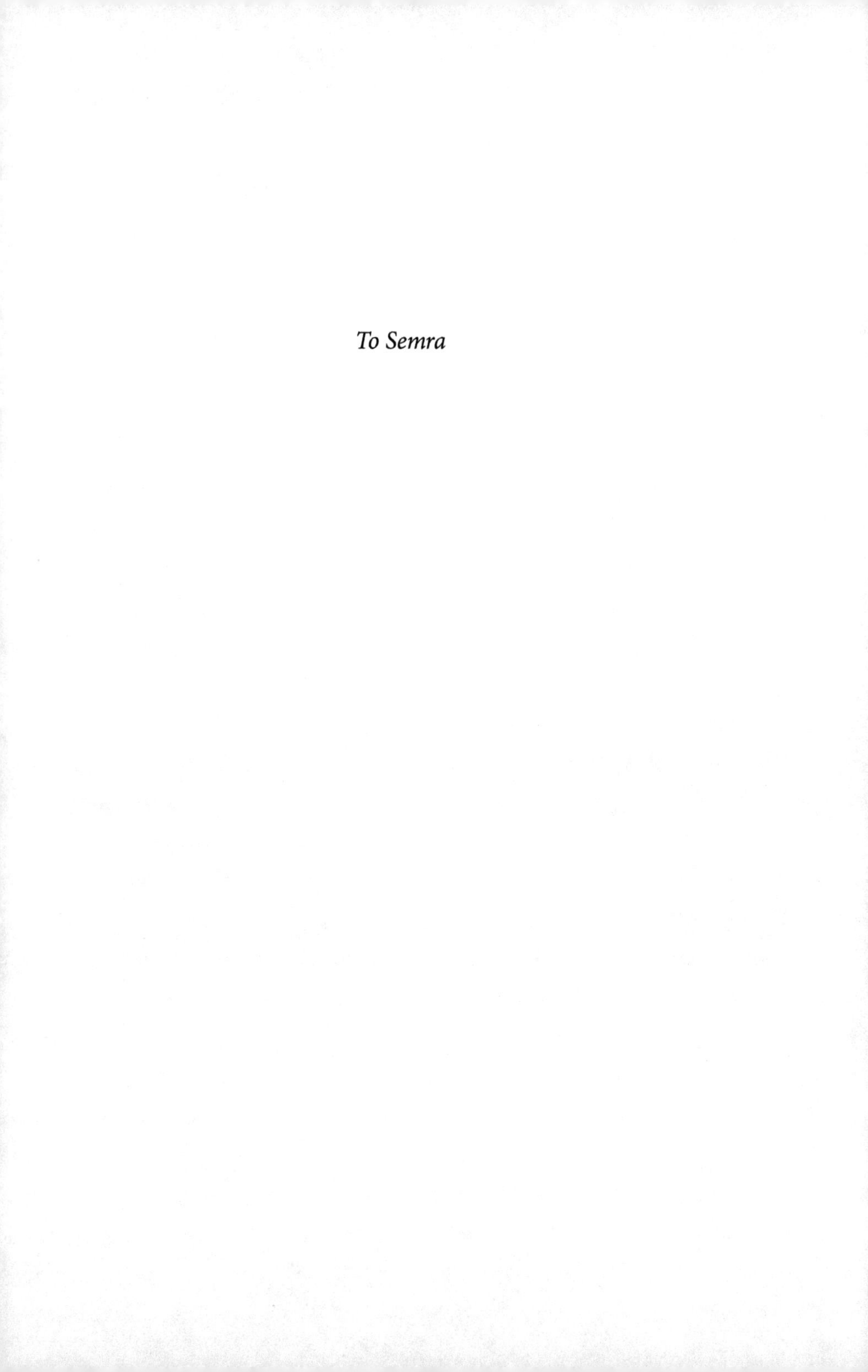

To Semra

Acknowledgements

This collection, as well as the taxing fieldwork on whose findings it stands are deeply indebted to a long list of individuals and institutions. Without their tireless efforts and support, neither the demanding research project nor the resulting volume could have seen the daylight.

First and foremost, I would like to express our deep gratitude to The Willows International Foundation (formerly Willows Foundation) for originating a research project to rigorously evaluate their reproductive health education programs in Ghana, Pakistan, Tanzania, and Turkey. Generous is too simple a word for doing justice to their financial sponsorship and administrative and intellectual guidance of the project from the day of its conception.

Several individuals connected with Willows International contributed to this effort at varying stages, but its founder, President, and CEO, *Dr. Türkiz Gökgöl*, was the powerful and driving engine behind it all. She was not only vitally instrumental in bringing the project to life but was an inspiration to all of us connected with the project.

The project proposal, with objectives, methodology, and technical details, was drawn up by Harvard University's T. H. Chan School of Public Health, which diligently administered the project, while *Dr. Iqbal H. Shah*, who is among the contributors of this volume, and *Dr. David Canning*, both of Harvard University, assumed the overall academic leadership of the design and implementation of the fieldwork. The whole team and I are greatly indebted to them and Harvard's School of Public Health.

In Turkey, Harvard University partnered with Bahçeşehir University in Istanbul. I cannot find the words to describe BAU's incredible support and encouragement at every phase of the project. Starting with *Mr. Enver Yücel*, the founder and Chair of the Board of Trustees of the University, down to officials at various positions, they have been unbelievably helpful. It is no exaggeration to say that, without Bahçeşehir University and its administrators, the Turkish leg of the project would not have been possible.

The fieldwork was carried out by SIA-Insight Research Firm. I would like to thank them and their CEO, *Mr. Hüseyin Tapinç*, for conducting all interviews meticulously and for double and sometimes even triple-checking every interview to assure the highest level of reliability possible.

Ms. Bahar Ayça Okçuoğlu and *Ms. Duygu Karadon*, both among contributors of this volume, were project managers who played an important role in bringing the fieldwork to a successful end. *Ms. Tuana Akbulut* skillfully and gleefully performed the tedious task of putting the manuscript in order, checking all references, numbering tables and figures and doing other essential chores.

Last but not least, I am deeply thankful to my wife *Semra* for patiently and cheerfully sharing the agony of yet another writing adventure of her toiling husband and for greatly contributing to the birth of this book.

Contents

About the Contributors

Dr. Yılmaz Esmer is professor at Bahçeşehir University, Istanbul, Turkey. He has been the principal investigator for Turkey of the World Values Surveys since 1990. He is also a member of the TRU (Transformation Research Unit) research team based at Stellenbosch University in S. Africa. He has recently completed the latest values survey in Turkey and is the principal investigator of the project on reproductive health and family planning in collaboration with T. H. Chan School of Public Health of Harvard University. He has published extensively on comparative values, political culture, religion and politics, democratization, electoral behavior and, more recently, on political and affective polarization.

Dr. Sarah Huber-Krum completed a post-doctoral fellowship for the Willows Impact Evaluation Project at Harvard University's School of Public Health. Dr. Huber-Krum holds a PhD in Social Work, and an MSW and MPA from The Ohio State University. Her research focuses on global sexual and reproductive health, specifically the contributing factors to contraceptive nonuse and contraceptive decision making within social and structural contexts. She has collaborated on projects located in Malawi, Tanzania, Ghana, India, Nepal, Sri Lanka, Turkey, Pakistan and the U.S.

Duygu Karadon is a research assistant at Bahçeşehir University Center for Economic and Social Research (BETAM), Istanbul, Turkey. She received her B.A. in Sociology (Bahçeşehir University), M.A. in Sociology (Mimar Sinan Fine Arts University, Istanbul), and a second M.A. in Cinema-Television (Bahçeşehir University). She directed the fieldwork for the Turkish Values Survey (part of the World Values Survey, wave-7). She was the Senior Project Assistant and Project Manager for the "Implementation and Impact Evaluation of the Willows' Reproductive Health Programs in Ghana, Pakistan, Tanzania, and Turkey" (in cooperation with Harvard T. H. Chan School of Public Health). Her research interests include cultural studies, comparative values, electoral behavior, social stratification, and survey methodology.

Bahar Ayça Okçuoğlu is a doctoral candidate in Sociology at Koç University, Istanbul, Turkey. After completing her bachelor's degree in Sociology at Bahçeşehir University, she continued her studies at London School of Economics and Political Science where she received master's degree in European Studies. She worked as a research assistant at Bahçeşehir University's Center for Economic and Social Research for 5 years actively participating in several projects. Her academic interests include cultural values, identity and diaspora studies, and particularly Circassian diaspora.

Dr. Julia Katherine Rohr is an Epidemiologist and Research Scientist at the Harvard T.H. Chan School of Public Health. She has led research projects on the Post-Partum IUD Impact Evaluation study in Tanzania and the Willows Reproductive Health Impact Evaluation project in Turkey. She is currently the Project Director for the Health and Aging in Africa: A Longitudinal Study of an INDEPTH Community in South Africa (HAALSI) project. Dr. Rohr's background is in HIV treatment and sexual behavior. She holds a PhD in Epidemiology from Boston University, where she worked as a data analyst and project manager at the Center for Global Health and Development at the BU School of Public Health for studies in Kenya, South Africa and Uganda.

Dr. Ryoko Sato is a research associate at Harvard T.H. Chan School of Public Health and at Center for Health Decision Science. She is a development economist, interested in identifying barriers to and incentives for health behaviors in developing countries. She received a Ph.D. in Economics from University of Michigan in 2015. Her research focuses on three main areas: (1) Impact evaluation of health interventions on changes in health behaviors and outcomes through rigorous causal studies such as randomized controlled trials; (2) Evaluation of determinants of health behaviors, outcomes, and disparities; and (3) Cost-effectiveness analysis of health interventions.

Dr. Iqbal H. Shah is a Principal Research Scientist in the Department of Global Health and Population at the Harvard T. H. Chan School of Public Health. He was the Principal Investigator of two multi-country studies: (1) Studying the Impact and Performance of Institutionalizing Immediate Postpartum IUD Services as a Routine Part of Antenatal Counselling and Delivery Room Services in Nepal, Sri Lanka and Tanzania; and (2) Implementation and Impact Evaluation of the Willows' Reproductive Health Programs in Ghana, Pakistan, Tanzania, and Turkey. From 1985 to 2012, Dr. Shah worked in the Department of Reproductive Health and Research (RHR) and the Special Programme in Human Reproduction (HRP) at the World Health Organization (WHO) in Geneva, Switzerland. At WHO, Dr. Shah was responsible for research and research capacity-building activities in Social Science and Operations Research in sexual and reproductive health and coordinating the team on Preventing

Unsafe Abortion. In 2016, he received *The Marjorie C. Horn Operations Research Award* from USAID in recognition of dedicated efforts "to building the capacity of social science researchers in developing countries, generating and utilizing research for policy development, and improving the lives of women and girls through better access to reproductive health care".

Dr. Rahime Süleymanoğlu-Kürüm is an associate professor in the Department of Political Science and International Relations at Bahçeşehir University. She is also an associate member of the Nottingham Interdisciplinary Centre for Economic and Political Research (NICEP). Her research focusses on Europeanization, EU foreign policy, Turkish foreign policy, gendering EU studies, gender and diplomacy and elite sociology. She is the author of *Conditionality, the EU and Turkey: From Transformation to Retrenchment* (Routledge, 2019) and co-editor of *Feminist Framing of Europeanisation: Gender Equality Policies in Turkey and the EU* (Palgrave Macmillan, 2021). Her scholarly articles have been published in prestigious journals such as *Political Studies Review* and *Geopolitics*.

YILMAZ ESMER

1 Introduction

1 An Ambitious Research Project

This book results from a challenging but rewarding collaborative research project between Harvard University's School of Public Health and Bahçeşehir University. The fieldwork carried out in Istanbul was part of a larger design that, in addition to Turkey, included Ghana, Pakistan, and Tanzania. The project took off in 2017 and was concluded in 2020. The research design was meticulously crafted in a series of meetings in Boston under the coordination of Dr. Iqbal H. Shah and Dr. David Canning, both of Harvard University, and with the active participation of principal investigators and collaborators from all partner institutions as well as from the funding agency.

The main objective of the project was to evaluate the impact of education programs targeting women's reproductive health initiated and sponsored by Willows International – a nonprofit organization aiming to expand the "utilization of comprehensive reproductive health services by providing individualized information, education, counseling, and referrals to women in communities in need of such services."[1]

Willows International launched its first program in Turkey in 1999 with enthusiastic support from the Ministry of Health and full cooperation of local authorities. The program's main objective in Turkey and all countries covered was to educate women of reproductive age about family planning and reproductive health. The present book focuses on Turkey, and the fieldwork carried out in Istanbul.[2] However, before analyzing the findings from the fieldwork, we first provide a brief background about the cultural and political setting in the country.

The empirical component of the project was quite comprehensive and included household, facility, exit, and pharmacy surveys and key informant interviews. For the household survey (also referred to as the baseline survey), the plan was to interview one woman of reproductive age (ages 16–44) in each selected household. The sites chosen were the districts of Bağcılar (Willows intervention site) and Küçükçekmece (comparison site), both in Istanbul. A total of 4,224 household interviews (2,112 in each site) were completed, providing satisfactory coverage of the target population, given that there were a total of 23,099 households at the intervention site and 14,981 households at the control site.

The details of the household sample are shown in Fig. 1.1. Data collection for the baseline household survey occurred between March 27 and June 27, 2018. Interviews were conducted by an all-women team of experienced interviewers who completed a week-long training program led by a team of Harvard, BAU, and SIA-Insight experts.

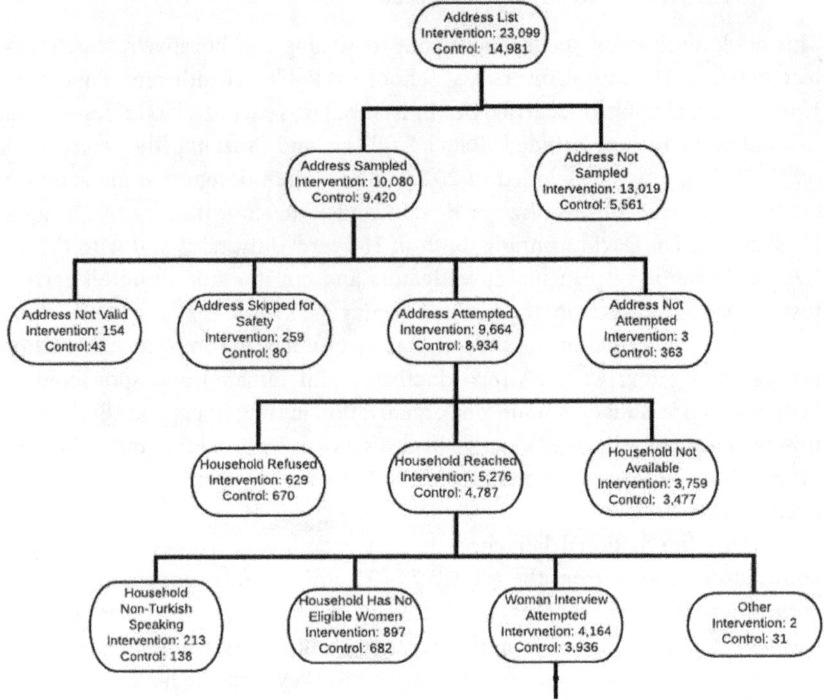

Fig. 1.1: Sampling details for the household survey. The chart was prepared by D. Karadon, B. A. Okçuoğlu, and J. K. Rohr.

Household interviews were complemented with 35 neighborhood health facility surveys and 311 exit interviews. The team also conducted 126 pharmacy surveys (including 26 pharmacies and 100 shops). Finally, 16 key informant interviews with community stakeholders (8) and family planning providers (8) were completed.

A total of 40 health care facilities at both the intervention and control sites were targeted in collaboration with the Istanbul Office of Willows International. Data collection was completed in 35 of these 40 health facilities. (Of the remaining five, one was no longer in existence; two were no longer providing family planning services, and there were only two refusals.) Thus, the project intended to cover every major dimension of female reproductive health with data collected from all actors involved in the process.

By the end of 2019, all data collection had been completed, and the teams were set for analyses, which are reported in the present volume and numerous articles authored by team members and published in various scholarly journals. For a list of published bibliographies on the project, we refer the reader to Chapter 4.

Much more detailed information about the basic approach and the project's design is given in Chapter 4 by Iqbal H. Shah.

2 Plan of the Book

The two chapters in Part One are intended to give the reader a background on Turkey's overall cultural and political structures related to family planning and reproductive health. It is hoped that the national perspective of these two chapters will help the reader place our findings in a broader context.

The first of these two chapters (Chapter 2) by Yılmaz Esmer draws from a recent nationwide values survey to investigate the association between cultural values, norms, attitudes and behavior, and attitudes related to family planning in the Turkish context. The survey instrument includes many questions that are asked globally in the latest round of the World Values Surveys[3] and several Turkey-specific value questions plus knowledge, behavior, and attitude questions on family planning and contraception. The key independent variables that impact fertility behavior and preferences analyzed are religiosity and religious values, political ideology, gender roles and materialistic/post-materialistic values. Of these independent variables, religiosity and religious values seem to deserve particular attention – a finding that is not surprising in a predominantly Muslim society.

Chapter 3, authored by Rahime Süleymanoğlu-Kürüm, analyzes family planning policies in Turkey with particular attention to political and ideological polarization. This perspective enables the reader to gain a deeper understanding of the changing policies that parallel the political developments in the country and their root causes. The chapter is rich in historical data going back to the founding year of the Republic and thus serves as a reference for those interested in sketching the development of family planning policies in Turkey. However, limiting our summary to family planning policies would not be fair to the author. Perhaps even more interestingly, we find in Süleymanoğlu-Kürüm's article an analysis of the changes in the perception of women concerning their societal roles. This, I believe, makes the chapter a stimulating read not only for those focusing mainly on family planning and reproductive health issues in particular but also for a wider audience interested in women's studies and feminism. As the author writes, Chapter 3 "sets the ground for the empirical analysis to be presented in the subsequent chapters of the volume." And, as the editor of the volume, I might add that it does an excellent job of doing so.

The six chapters in Part Two report and analyze the methodology, and the major findings of the field study are briefly referred to in this Introduction.

Chapter 4 by Iqbal H. Shah provides a detailed account of the project's design that was similarly implemented in Ghana, Pakistan, Tanzania, and Turkey. From a methodological perspective, the study, as a whole, used state-of-the-art techniques that included both quantitative and qualitative components. Shah's article explains both the quantitative (household interviews of women of child-bearing age, exit interviews conducted at facilities that provide family planning services) and qualitative (in-depth interviews with health care providers and various community stakeholders) aspects of the study, thus helping the reader gain a full grasp of project methodology. Chapter 4 provides the framework for interpreting the data skillfully analyzed in the following chapters.

In Chapter 5, Duygu Karadon delineates the association between sociocultural factors and decisions and preferences related to contraception and induced abortion. Chapter 2 offers a more general and national framework for analyzing this association, while Karadon's article gives us a rich and focused analysis using the project's data. Through in-depth interviews, data are collected from family planning service providers and community stakeholders. This qualitative study, which complements the quantitative chapters in a meaningful way, again underlines religiosity's prominence as an independent variable. Gender roles, particularly within the family, emerge as another factor that should not be ignored in understanding contraceptive and family planning decisions.

The following chapter, Chapter 6, by Sarah Huber-Krum, brings a remarkably interesting perspective to the book. It is often argued, and I believe justifiably so, that the present-day Turkish society is beleaguered by two major cultural and political fault lines: the secular-religious divide and the ethnic (i.e., Turkish-Kurdish) divide. Sarah-Krum's article tackles the ethnic fault line, exploring the impact of Turkish/Kurdish identity on the choice of contraceptives. Based on a random sample of 3,038 married women of reproductive age, her analysis suggests that those whose self-reported identity is Kurdish are more likely to use modern contraceptive methods. This outcome is somewhat contradictory to the widely shared assumption. Huber-Krum explains this unexpected finding, hypothesizing that the difference between the two ethnic identities might be due to the duration of residence in Istanbul. Put differently, the length of stay in a metropolis such as Istanbul might be more significant than ethnicity.

Chapter 7 by Bahar Ayça Okçuoğlu and Sarah Huber-Krum focuses on women's empowerment and underlines the fact that, in addition to historical, political, and economic circumstances, "women's attitudes and values may be important determinants of their reproductive health behaviors." It is argued that women's empowerment and relative autonomy – no doubt closely related to cultural factors such as conservative values and religiosity – must also be considered to reach a full understanding of women's reproductive behavior. The authors employ several sophisticated quantitative methods to assess the relative importance of empowerment, autonomy, conservative values, and religiosity. Parallel to the findings of the other chapters and several unrelated studies, their main conclusion is that religious values (in addition to the level of education) are the main determinants of contraceptive behavior.

In Chapter 8, Ryoko Sato introduces another interesting perspective to our data. She analyzes the effects of distance to a health facility – obviously a significant factor in deciding to utilize the services provided – on family planning. Perhaps not unexpected but certainly worthy of consideration is her main conclusion: "The effect of distance to a health facility on contraceptive use significantly differs according to family planning availability at the health facility." Equally important is the distinction Sato makes between long-acting and short-acting family planning. We learn that the effects of distance are not similar on these two categories of decisions. In one sentence, Sato's article is interesting and sophisticated academically and contains invaluable suggestions for policy-makers.

In the concluding chapter (Chapter 9), Julia Katherine Rohr first gives a descriptive account of the level of knowledge related to contraception and of different methods available to couples. Also important are the sources of this knowledge. The next question Rohr confronts is the reason – or reasons – behind the choice of method and its frequency of use. The factors that impact the choice between modern, long-acting, reversible methods and traditional methods are of particular significance. With its more general approach and analyses, Chapter 9 thus serves as an overall conclusion to our volume.

Notes

1. https://www.willowsintl.org/about-us; accessed 5 July 2021.
2. Editor of the present volume, Yılmaz Esmer of Bahçeşehir University in Istanbul, was the principal investigator of the Turkish project from its planning stages to its conclusion. Bahar Ayca Okçuoglu and Duygu Karadon, both of

whom contributed articles to this volume, planned and supervised the day-to-day tasks and ensured that the fieldwork adhered to the highest standards of quality. Sevval Simay Baykal and Sebahat Kurutaş assisted the project at every stage of its implementation as well as taking active part in interviews and other aspects of the fieldwork. SIA-Insight, an Istanbul based and highly reputed research firm, was responsible for the recruitment and organization of interviewers, trained jointly by a team of Harvard and Bahçeşehir researchers. SIA-Insight also took responsibility for routine fieldwork and data collection.
3. For more information on World Values Surveys, refer to www.worldvaluessurvey.org.

Part One Culture and Politics of Fertility Behavior: The National Perspective

YILMAZ ESMER

2 Cultural Values, Reproductive Health and Family Planning: The Turkish Case

Abstract: This chapter uses data from a nationwide survey of values and fertility behavior. Hence, it analyzes the association between values, norms and ideology on attitudes and behavior concerning family planning and contraception. Particular attention is paid to religious values, political ideology, conservatism/liberalism and materialistic/post-materialistic variables, and gender equity as independent variables to assess their impact on attitudes and behavior related to fertility preferences and use of contraceptives. Determinants of contraceptive method choice (modern vs. traditional) are also analyzed in detail.

Keywords: Cultural values, family planning, contraception, fertility behavior.

Turkey is very fortunate with respect to the availability of high-quality, nationwide time-series demographic survey data which goes back more than half a century. Thanks to the efforts of few visionaries and productive international collaboration, the Hacettepe Institute of Population Studies (HIPS) of Hacettepe University was founded in 1967. One of the main missions of HIPS, from the very start, was to "to conduct surveys analyzing the demographic, social, economic, cultural and medical aspects of population studies" (2019).[1] Almost immediately after its founding, HIPS conducted its first demographic survey in 1968, using state-of-the-art methodology and providing invaluable data on reproductive behavior and attitudes as well as wider demographic topics and family structure. Albeit under different labels, HIPS has continued the series and the latest "Turkish Demographic and Health Survey" (TDHS) was carried out in 2018. Thus, both researchers and policy-makers now have access to reliable time-series data which spans over 52 years and comprises 11 nationwide surveys. This, indeed, is a formidable accomplishment in a developing country with rather limited research infrastructure especially in the 1970s and 1980s.

However, significant as they are, cultural values lie outside the scope of HIPS surveys which, quite understandably, do not include value questions. The primary source for Turkish society's values, attitudes, beliefs on a broad range of topics is the data collected by the Turkish values studies conducted as part of the European Values Study and World Values Surveys.[2]

Turkey joined the World Values Surveys, a longitudinal international survey program covering around 100 countries, back in 1990. World Values Surveys, carried out at roughly five-year intervals, aim at measuring all major value domains in all inhabited continents of the world. Turkey was part of every wave (to date, there have been seven waves of global surveys with the first one dating back to 1981) of the surveys since 1990 and the data from nationally representative samples – a treasure for researchers – is readily and freely available from the World Values Survey Association or the European Values Study.

This brief introduction about the two international survey programs is intended to underline the fact that data on both family planning behavior and attitudes as well as cultural values are available for a time span of many decades to researchers working on Turkey. Furthermore, these data allow international comparisons, thus helping us to evaluate the Turkish case from a wider comparative perspective. The problem, however, is that, to the best of my knowledge, these two spheres have never been brought together in a unified analytical model but have progressed along two independent tracks. What was acutely needed, then, was national survey data covering both reproductive health, behavior and attitudes as well as cultural values. This is of great importance since – as I shall try to demonstrate in the next section– we are well aware that reproductive behavior and attitudes are not independent of cultural values. To the contrary, research has evidenced that religious values are closely associated with, for instance, fertility behavior, approval and use of contraceptives, attitudes towards induced abortions, etc. Indeed, there is a wide-ranging literature on the association between religion, religious values, secularism and fertility behavior (for an extensive and recent review, see Galbraith & Shaver, 2018). Another largely researched topic within this tradition is the correlation between values related to gender, gender equity and fertility. To put it in more general terms, values which can be viewed under the umbrella of "liberal philosophy" are almost universally associated with higher levels of modern contraceptive use and, consequently, lower levels of total fertility.

1 Cultural Values and Reproductive Behavior: Correlation or Causality?

> *The mainstay of anthropological understanding of contraceptives at work is the concept of "culture", which pervades the forms and expressions of human agency, facilitating some and constraining others.*
>
> Russell & Thompson, 2000, p.1

We will be in distinguished company when we maintain that not only reproductive but any kind of behavior is, to some degree – and in many cases to a very large degree– explained by cultural values (Ellis & Thompson, 1997; Fukuyama, 1995; Harrison & Huntington, 2000; Hofstede, 2001; Inglehart, 1977, 1997; Inglehart & Norris, 2003; Inglehart & Baker, 2000; Inglehart & Welzel, 2005; Inkeles, 1983; Inkeles & Smith, 1974; Schwartz, 1996, 2006; Van de Kaa, 2001). This brief list of references could easily be extended to include great philosophers and scholars all the way from Plato and Aristotle to Ibn Khaldun, Montesquieu, J. S. Mill, de Tocqueville, Weber and others. But my aim in this chapter is to demonstrate the, hopefully causal, link between cultural values and reproductive (fertility) behavior in contemporary Turkey.

To begin analyzing the association between values and fertility behavior, the first question that needs to be addressed is the identification of relevant cultural values that will help to explain the variance in behavior.

I have already referred above to the bibliography on "religion and fertility behavior" which includes the published entries on the subject and which is about 250 pages long. And I suspect this is only part – albeit the most significant part– of the publications to be found in all corners of the globe and in several languages. On the other hand, this is only natural since every major – and perhaps minor, as well– religion has something to say about human sexuality, reproduction, marriage and family life in general. In fact, monotheist religions have rather strict lists of do's and do not's on these aspects of human existence. It would not be an exaggeration to say that monotheist religions were concerned and pre-occupied with human sexuality more than any other aspect of human behavior.

Research seems to indicate that both religion (particular faith that one identifies with)[3] and religiosity (level of observance of religious principles and teachings) have an impact on reproductive behavior. Not surprisingly, religiosity effect is found to be stronger than religion effect. (Dean & Shaver, 2018; Schnabel, 2021; Thornton, 2005; Allendorf & Thornton, 2015; Thornton et al., 2015). It is also worth noting that the religion effect on fertility behavior is not uniform across all societies and that these effects subside with economic development. Thus, while in Nigeria, for example, religion and ethnicity are extremely significant in shaping reproductive behavior (Obasohan, 2015), in the United States, fertility rates of Catholics and Protestants have now all but converged (Galbraith & Shaver, 2018). Indeed, Obasohan (2015, Table 1) reports that in Nigeria, a multi-ethnic and multi-religion society, while only 5.6 % of Muslim women of reproductive age report using any contraceptive at all, the corresponding figures for Catholics is 25.8 % and other Christians 26.4 %, respectively. Also globally true is the fact that people not affiliated with any religion and atheists/agnostics tend to have much lower total fertility rates than the faithful (Schnabel, 2021).

The examples above (and the list of case studies with similar findings) can be expanded considerably but the point is clear: both religious affiliation or non-affiliation and degree of religiosity of individuals are closely associated with reproductive behavior although the impact of the former decreases in magnitude in developed nations.

A rather additional and interesting note is that secularism is closely correlated with fertility not only at the individual but also aggregate level. Put differently, average secularism levels of countries have strong bearing on both total fertility rates of countries and also on individuals' fertility behavior (Schnabel, 2021).

In addition to religion and religiosity, an important set of variables related to reproductive behavior are attitudes concerning gender issues in general and gender equity in particular. According to Arpino, Esping-Andersen and Pessin (2013, p. 13) "The more women and men agree on equitable values, the more 'dramatic' is the transition in the sense that its effects are more evident on fertility." Schnabel (2021) explains the link between secularism and fertility by introducing women's autonomy as an intervening variable. Said differently, according to Schnabel, secularism gives rise to more liberal values concerning gender equity and, at least partially, this is the mechanism that accounts for lower fertility rates in more secular countries. In his words:

> Secular countries promote greater autonomy for women, their lives, and their bodies. But more religious countries tend to have cultural values – familism, drive to family formation, idealized fertility, and even explicit injunctions to "be fruitful and multiply" – that promote pronatalist preferences, a reluctance to use modern contraceptives and abortion, and generally greater control over women, their lives, and their bodies. (Schnabel, 2021, p. 14)

I have already referred to the importance of so-called "liberal values" (i.e. value domains other than religiosity and gender roles) in explaining the variances in especially modern contraceptive use and, relatedly, total fertility rates. These, for the most part, correspond to what Inglehart and Welzel (2005), Welzel (2010), and Inglehart (2018) have called self-expression values.

Of necessity, I am forced to limit the number of independent variables whose effects on fertility are to be tested. Consequently, from among the long list of self-expression values, I have chosen those which I believe will be more significant for the purposes of this chapter. These are: tolerance of "the others," control over one's life (versus fatalism), and tolerance of different sexual orientations.

Before proceeding with statistical analyses, it may be worth reiterating my theoretical perspective. The theoretical question is whether it is socio-economic structure or culture that accounts for more of the variation in fertility and related variables such as the acceptance of the use of modern contraceptives. There is no doubt that both of these should have significant effects. Equally certain is the fact that socio-economic structural variables and cultural values are, in most instances, closely correlated. Nevertheless, as explained in the beginning, I maintain that cultural factors have at least equal, if not greater, impact on reproductive behavior. With respect to religion, Galbraith and Shaver (2018) trace these two approaches to Marx and Weber.

With this background in mind, we are now ready to proceed with describing our data and identifying our variables to be analyzed.

2 Data and Variables

The present Chapter, as the rest of the book, focuses on Turkey and, consequently, Turkish data. Thus, the analyses in this Chapter are based on data from a nationwide survey (n = 2,401) of Turkey, using a full probability multi-stage sample of all residents age 18 and over and covering no less than 68 out of Turkey's 81 provinces. The questionnaire comprised a wide range of value questions[4] and a number of questions designed to tap the attitudes and behavior related to reproductive health and family planning. The mode of data collection was face-to-face interviewing. Many of our reproductive health and family planning questions are the same or very similar to the ones used in the most recent TDHS. Data collection took place from March to May 2018.

Our main task, of course, is to delineate the relationships between these two clusters of variables. Put differently, we would like to analyze in detail the relationship between cultural value domains and reproductive behavior and preferences.

2.1 Dependent Variables

The dependent variables used in the analysis include both behavioral and attitudinal aspects of fertility and family planning. Explained briefly, these are:

a. *Total fertility:* The relevance of this variable needs no elaboration. Following Lakomy (2017), only women over 40 and men over 50 are used in analyses with this variable to exclude women and men who have not completed their fertility. This cut-off point for women can be justified by the findings of the most recent Turkey Demographic and Health Survey (Hacettepe University Institute of Population Studies, 2019).[5] Needless to say, this restriction limits the sample size for analyses of total fertility rather significantly.

b. *Knowledge of modern contraceptives*: This variable measures respondents' knowledge of contraceptive methods. Thus, I calculate the total number of modern contraceptive methods, over the ten modern methods asked,[6] that the respondent knows or has ever heard about. The survey showed that, in our sample of 2,401 respondents, 275 (14.0%) is not aware of even a single method. On the other hand, the proportion of those who claim to have heard of eight, nine or all ten methods mentioned is 17.8%. The youngest age group (18–24) seems to be somewhat less knowledgeable than the older respondents and the regression coefficient for age has a statistically significant effect on this variable (Tab. 2.2).
c. *Preference for a traditional method*: According to the most recent TDHS, 20% of married women of reproductive age (15–49) use withdrawal for birth control. By way of comparison, in our survey, the proportion of women who reported using withdrawal among those who currently use any method was found to be 19.7% while the comparable figure for men was 16.9%. The dependent variable (dichotomous) I use in the analysis is expressed preference (actual or hypothetical) for withdrawal again among women and men who currently use family planning (26% expressed this preference).
d. *Attitude towards abortion*: This variable measures approval of induced abortions on a scale of 1 to 10 where 1 indicates "totally unjustified" and 10 denotes "completely justified." Although legal, under certain conditions, in Turkey since 1983, there is still a sizeable population which strongly disapproves of induced abortions. This attitude is strongly encouraged by the pronatalist preferences and policies of the religiously conservative Justice and Development Party (AKP) which has been in power since 2002. The arithmetic mean of our 10-point scale is 2.58, that is, very close to the total disapproval end of the scale. Additionally, fully 56% of the sample scored 1 on the scale, i.e. the strongest disapproval score possible.
e. *Approval of induced abortion for unwanted child*: The last independent variable analyzed defines more specific conditions under which induced abortions may be approved: This is another dichotomous variable (1 approve; 2 disapprove) intended to measure the prevalence of what could described as the most liberal attitude towards abortion – basically saying "I simply want to terminate this pregnancy" is sufficient justification.

2.2 Independent Variables

The independent variables described below aim to cover all noteworthy domains in the values and fertility literature that I have very briefly referred to above. Religiosity (of course, in Turkey, an almost exclusively Islamic society, religion is a constant) and attitudes concerning gender roles and gender equity appear as the two most significant value spheres that one should pay close attention to. Also found significant in various studies are liberal values (e.g. tolerance) and political ideology. Clearly, this is not an exhaustive list of possible predictors but I believe they will suffice for the purpose of this chapter.

To measure religiosity, I use three indicators, two of which are conventional and used frequently in numerous surveys. The third measure is by the present author and is intended for Turkey and perhaps other Islamic societies.

Values taken as indicators of gender equity and especially the position of women vis-à-vis that of men is an additive scale of eight survey questions.

In short, I use the following explanatory variables in the analyses:

a. *Importance of God:* This is a 10-point scale asking about the importance of God in respondent's life and has been used in values questionnaires, including World Values Surveys and European Values Study, for decades.
b. *Mosque attendance*: Frequency of formal attendance in religious services is another conventional indicator of religiosity. Our question had seven response categories ranging from more than weekly to never or almost never attendance. It should be noted that, unlike most other religions, in Sunni Islam, mosque attendance is obligatory only for men.
c. *Women's swimsuit*: This indicator, first introduced by Esmer, seems to have worked well in numerous surveys as a significant predictor of voting behavior, political preferences, religious observance, etc. (see, for example, Esmer, 2002a). It is inspired by the observation that "The cultural gap separating Islam from the West involves Eros far more than Demos." (Norris & Inglehart, 2002, p. 236). Esmer (2002b, p. 297) reached a similar conclusion with respect to the defining characteristic of Islamic civilizations: "… very significant characteristic of Islamic culture is its outlook on women and sex." Consequently, Islamic populations are sensitive about displaying female physique in public. Thus, the question I ask is whether or not the respondent thinks women's wearing swimsuit on the beach is a sin.
d. *Gender equity*: An additive index of gender equity was constructed with the following eight items all of which ranged between 1 (completely agree) and 4 (completely disagree).
    i. When a mother works for pay, the children suffer.
    ii. On the whole, men make better political leaders then women do.
    iii. University education is more important for a boy than a girl.
    iv. On the whole, men make better business executives than women do.
    v. Being a housewife is just as fulfilling as working for pay.
    vi. In our society, it is more fitting for men to be the head of household.
    vii. Some women deserve to be beaten by their husbands.

viii. A wife should always obey her husband and do as he tells her.

The first five items are taken from WVS/EVS questionnaires while the last three are specific to this survey. The scale has rather high reliability with a Cronbach's Alpha of 0.82.

e. *Political ideology:* This item, tapping respondent's self-placement on a 10-point left-right scale is also taken from WVS/EVS (and a number of other) questionnaires with a score of 1 indicating extreme left and 10 denoting extreme right.
f. *Tolerance:* As commented above, tolerance is an important liberal value shown to be associated with fertility behavior. On the other hand, acceptance of "unorthodox" sexual orientations is an important trait of postmaterialism (Inglehart & Welzel, 2005). With this consideration in mind, I use a 10-point justification of homosexuality scale. I would like to remind the reader that Turkey traditionally has had one of the lowest levels of tolerance for homosexuality among all countries surveyed by WVS.
g. *Traditional vs Modern outlook:* An important characteristic of traditional cultures is a strong belief in pre-determinism or fate. On the other hand, "modern" individual is thought to believe to have full control over his/her life. The variable used in the following analyses is a 10-point fatalism/free will scale with the lower extreme indicating a belief that life is totally predetermined by fate and the upper end representing individuals claiming complete control over their lives.

2.3 Control Variables

The following control variables are used in all regressions:

a. *Level of education*: No formal schooling; primary school diploma; secondary school diploma; college education or above.
b. *Age*: Year of interview minus respondent's year of birth.
c. *Income group*: 10 income groups from lowest to highest.
d. *Financial satisfaction*: Subjective evaluation of respondent's degree of satisfaction the financial situation of his/her household (a 10-point scale).
e. *Gender:* Male or female.

3 Results: Values or Structure or Both?

It will be noticed that I will be analyzing a longer than usual list of dependent variables (actually, the list could be even longer but this is only a chapter, not a book). The reason for this is the desire to include as many important aspects of reproductive behavior and attitudes as is feasible. Thus, the following analyses cover behavior, knowledge and attitudes related to fertility. To assess the impact of independent and control variables, I use OLS for dependent variables that are – or can reasonably be treated as– interval level and binary logistic regression in the case of dichotomous dependent variables. Tables 2.1 to 2.5 summarize the findings, i.e. relevant coefficients. However, in order to avoid unnecessary details and even confusion, variables whose statistical significance level exceed 0.05 have been omitted from the tables.

Starting with Tab. 2.1 where total fertility is the dependent variable, most of the signs are in the expected direction except for two. Religious values indeed have a sizeable impact on total fertility with three indicators of religiosity all being highly significant. However, mosque attendance behaves in a rather curious fashion and stands apart from the two other indicators. In short, those who believe women's wearing swim suit is a sin and those who attach more importance to God in their lives tend to have higher levels of fertility. This finding is totally in line with the existing literature which I have briefly referred to above. In addition, "first prize" goes to the swim suit variable which has the highest standardized coefficient (beta) among not only religiosity but all seven independent variables of significance. However, one is hard pressed to explain why mosque attendance behaves differently with a negative impact on fertility. (Please note that higher values of that variable indicate less, not more frequent attendance.). The answer to this puzzle probably lies in the fact that, as mentioned above, women are not required to attend weekly Friday prayers and most usually do not.[7] Unfortunately, leaving out women from the equation reduces sample size considerably and is therefore not very meaningful.

Again, it is not surprising that our "gender equality index" has a negative impact on total fertility. Recalling that the items that make up this index have a reliability score of 0.82, we can safely argue that all indicators of positive attitudes towards women's rights, equality, and independence result in reduced total fertility.

Of the demographic and economic indicators, age has a positive and level of satisfaction with household's financial situation a negative impact on total fertility. With total fertility rates in steady decline, it is only natural that older generations have higher levels of fertility. What is not so expected is the positive effect of household income. This is rather unexpected indeed.

Variables excluded from Tab. 2.1 seem to be as interesting as those included. One such variable of obvious interest is the level of education. While it may be speculated that this is due to the presumed high correlation between education and attitudinal independent variables, this is not the case. The strongest association of education is with our gender equity index and even that correlation (Pearson's r) is a meager 0.14.

From Tab. 2.1, one conclusion is clear: values related to religiosity and gender equity are at least as important as demography and economics.

Tab. 2.1: Determinants of total fertility (stepwise OLS; $p \leq .05$)

Predictor variables	**b**	**St. error of b**	**Beta**	**t**	**Sig.**
Constant	1.62	0.68		2.39	0.017
Women's swimsuit a sin	−0.65	0.13	−0.24	−5.12	0.000
Monthly income group	0.12	0.04	0.13	3.01	0.003
Satisfaction with financial situation of household	−0.07	0.03	−0.11	−2.42	0.016
Age	0.02	0.01	0.12	2.75	0.006
Frequency of mosque attendance	0.09	0.03	0.13	2.81	0.005
Gender equity index	−0.04	0.01	−0.12	−2.79	0.006
Importance of God scale	0.06	0.03	0.09	1.98	0.049
$r^2 = 0.14$; adjusted $r^2 = 0.13$					

Table 2.2 reports the statistically significant predictors of knowledge of modern contraceptives (i.e. 10 methods named in Note 6). It is apparent that significant predictors of knowledge are somewhat different from those of behavior (Tab. 2.1). However, this should not come as a surprise since the dependent variable is not at all related to behavior or attitude but rather just information. Clearly, then, education, age and monthly income would increase level of knowledge and they indeed do. Given that in Turkey contraception is regarded mainly as a female responsibility, the gender effect is also in the expected direction. Of the two attitudinal variables, we observe the positive impact of tolerance for homosexuality. But why should the more religious – as measured by the importance of God variable– be more knowledgeable about modern contraceptives? In a perhaps at best partially satisfactory answer to this question, we note that fertility behavior and knowledge of modern contraception are not correlated with each other. In fact, Pearson's r between these two variables is negative although it does not attain statistical significance in our sample.

Tab. 2.2: Determinants of level of knowledge of modern contraceptives (stepwise OLS; $p \leq .05$)

Predictor variables	b	St. error of b	Beta	t	Sig.
Constant	−4.24	0.60		−7.02	0.000
Importance of God scale	0.37	0.04	0.26	10.11	0.000
Tolerance for homosexuality scale	0.39	0.04	0.23	9.02	0.000
Monthly income group	0.28	0.05	0.14	5.15	0.000
Gender	0.87	0.16	0.14	5.62	0.000
Level of schooling	0.33	0.09	0.10	3.60	0.000
Age	0.02	0.01	0.09	3.19	0.001
$r^2 = 0.17$; adjusted $r^2 = 0.17$					

Table 2.3 evaluates preference for the most common traditional method, withdrawal as the dependent variable. It is a binary variable and therefore is analyzed using logistic regression. It will be observed that only four independent variables attain statistical significance and three of them are value related. Briefly, as religiosity, measured by mosque attendance (recall that it is coded in reverse) and women's swimsuit variables, increases, preference for withdrawal increases as well. The same is true for age which increases the odds of preferring this traditional method. These results are to be expected. However, the effect of our gender equity index is in need of an explanation. Why should this index have a positive impact on the preference for withdrawal? One could argue that individuals who are more in favor of women's rights and gender equity are more likely to assign more responsibility to the male partner for contraception. However, this finding certainly calls for more detailed investigation.

It will be noticed that no demographic or economic variable other than age is included in Tab. 2.3. Once again, it is not the economy!

Tab. 2.3: Determinants of preference for the traditional method (withdrawal) (Logistic regression)

Predictor variables	b	St. error of b	Sig.	Exp(B)
Constant	−1.46	0.93	0.116	0.23
Mosque attendance	0.13	0.06	0.022	1.14
Women's swimsuit a sin (yes/no)	−0.77	0.21	0.000	0.46
Gender equity index	0.07	0.02	0.001	1.08
Age	0.02	0.01	0.010	1.02
Nagelkerke $r^2 = 0.12$				

Table 2.4 has a rather straightforward interpretation with no surprises – at least, as far as the variables that are included in the table are concerned. One could easily predict that (i) higher approval of homosexuality, (ii) stronger belief in individual control over one's life, and (iii) higher levels of support for women's rights and gender equity would result in higher levels of approval of abortion. Also, and as expected, higher income groups are more likely to believe that induced abortions are justified. On the other hand, those placing themselves more to the right of the ideology scale are, almost by definition, less likely to approve of induced abortions.

Another point that is noteworthy about Tab. 2.4 is the rather unusually high r^2 value. Indeed, the five independent variables explain nearly half of the variance in the abortion approval scale.

However, once again, the variables that do not reach significance are unexpected. By now, we have come to expect the weak effects of education but Tab. 2.4 leaves out all three of our religiosity indicators as well. Plus, age and gender also fail to perform as expected.

Tab. 2.4: Determinants of approval of abortion scale (higher values indicate stronger approval/justification) (stepwise OLS; $p \leq .05$)

Predictor variables	**b**	**St. error of b**	**Beta**	**t**	**Sig.**
Constant	−0.43	0.29		−1.49	0.137
Tolerance for homosexuality scale	0.70	0.02	0.62	31.44	0.000
Monthly income group	0.20	0.03	0.14	7.41	0.000
Fatalism/Free will scale	0.07	0.02	0.08	3.98	0.000
Left-Right ideology scale	−0.05	0.02	−0.06	−3.03	0.002
Gender equity index	0.02	0.01	0.04	2.24	0.025
$r^2 = 0.45$; adjusted $r^2 = 0.45$					

The previous dependent variable was about approval or justification of induced abortions in general. In other words, the question did not specify any conditions under which the respondent would approve or disapprove of abortion but rather tapped the degree of a broad, overall "liberal" attitude about abortion. Obviously, when answering this question, the respondent could well have in mind circumstances such as mother's life being in danger, the unborn baby having a serious, debilitating genetic disease, rape or a similarly serious concern. Therefore, being specific about the circumstances under which abortion will be carried out will be a better measure.

The dependent variable in Tab. 2.5 asks about approval of ending pregnancy simply when the child is unwanted. Thus, this question specifies the most lenient circumstances. Its approval would certainly mean approval of abortion under more compelling situations. As shown in Tab. 2.5, rightist ideology significantly increases the odds of disapproval of ending an unwanted pregnancy. Once again, this finding is nothing to write home about and is a universal characteristic of right wing/conservative ideology. The rest of the story is also quite parallel to approval of induced abortions in general as explained above.

Tab. 2.5: Determinants of approval of aborting an unwanted child (Logistic regression)

Predictor variables	b	St. error of b	Sig.	Exp(B)
Constant	5.43	0.73	0.000	228.57
Left-Right ideology scale	0.16	0.03	0.000	1.17
Gender equity index	−0.11	0.02	0.000	0.90
Tolerance for homosexuality scale	−0.27	0.04	0.000	0.77
Fatalism/Free will scale	−0.11	0.03	0.002	0.90
Income group	−0.32	0.05	0.000	0.72
Gender	0.41	0.15	0.009	1.50
Nagelkerke $r^2 = 0.27$				

4 Conclusion

The main research question I tried to tackle in this Chapter was concerned with the impact of values and attitudes – culture, if you will– on decisions and behavior related to fertility. The answer to this question seems to be simple and quite straightforward: culture matters and matters a lot. This finding is in complete agreement with existing literature and goes to show that Turkey is not an exception to the rule.

The dependent variables analyzed include behavior (total fertility), knowledge (awareness of modern methods of contraception) as well as attitudinal indicators (approval of abortion in general and under more specific circumstances; preference for traditional contraception). On the other hand, in agreement with the existing literature very briefly reviewed above, predictor variables included in regression analyses focus on religiosity, women's rights and gender equity, tolerance, and political ideology. Needless to say, all common controls (e.g. income, education, age, gender) were taken into account as well.

Of the regressions reported, there is not a single one which does not include more than one cultural variable whose effects are highly significant, usually to the order of p being less than one in ten thousand. However, no single predictor attains significance in all equations. This is to be expected since dependent variables measure a wide range of concepts.

Other than the fact that values play an important role in determining various aspects of fertility behavior and preferences, some additional and interesting findings emerge. In a nutshell,

- Religious values are extremely important in determining total fertility as well as knowledge and choice of contraceptives. Interestingly, this is not true for abortion related variables. It seems like abortion approval in Turkey is somewhat weakly correlated with religiosity.
- Our composite gender index seems to work rather well indicating that gender attitudes play an important role in fertility behavior.
- Regarding women's swimsuit as a sin – an indicator both of religiosity and women's position in an Islamic society- is well– worth including in analyses of fertility behavior in addition to political and some other spheres.
- Higher tolerance for homosexuality is of significance for approval of induced abortions. This is perhaps due to the fact that, as emphasized in materialism-postmaterialism literature, this is an important indicator of so-called "self-expression values."

It is clear that demographic and economic variables are overshadowed by cultural indicators. In particular,

- One big surprise was the unexpectedly weak, and sometimes even non-existent, impact of level of education. This finding certainly merits further investigation, possibly with different measures of education such as years of schooling.
- Income, both objective and subjective, is also in need of additional analyses particularly in cases where it is not included in the equation.
- Of the two demographic variables, age has considerable impact and always in the expected direction. However, gender (male or female) is less important and the sign of its coefficients, where it enters the equation at all, are not straightforward to interpret.

I would like to conclude with one word of caution for policy-makers: Do not ignore or even underestimate the role played by cultural values on the outcome!

Notes

1. Although it was no doubt a team work, the heroic efforts of Professors Nusret Fişek and Frederic C. Shorter in the founding of the Institute as well as the launching of the first Turkish Demographic and Health Survey are gratefully acknowledged. Also worthy of mention is Prof. Serim Timur, whose seminal book on Turkish Family Structure (Timur 1972), based on data from the Institute's first survey, served as an indispensable reference for decades.
2. Detailed information about these two international survey programs can be found in their respective websites, www.worldvaluessurvey.org and www.europeanvaluesstudy.eu
3. For a useful and brief review of the basic teachings of major religions on contraceptive use, see Srikanthan and Reid (2008).
4. Value questions are basically taken from Wave 7 of the World Values Survey questionnaire with some country-specific questions relevant to our topic added.
5. Although, it would have been no doubt more preferable to raise the cutoff to 45 or 50 for women and 60 for men but this would have severely limited the sample size while having an almost completely negligible effect of the results.
6. Methods asked about are: female sterilization, male sterilization, pill, IUD, injectables, implant, condom, female condom, vaginal ring, and vaginal barrier methods (foam, gel, etc.)
7. On a 7-point scale of frequency of mosque attendance where higher values represent less frequent attendance, the mean for men is 2.95 and for women 4.52 – a considerable difference indeed.

References

Allendorf, K., & Thornton, A. (2015). Caste and choice: The influence of developmental idealism on marriage behavior. *American Journal of Sociology, 121*(1), 243–287.

Arpino, B., Esping-Andersen, G., & Pessin, L. (2013). The diffusion of gender egalitarian values and fertility. *Demo-Soc Working Paper, 51*. Retrieved April 3, 2021, from https://repositori.upf.edu/bitstream/handle/10230/22621/Arpino_Changes.pdf?sequence=3.

Ellis, R. J., & Thompson, M. (Eds.). (1997). *Culture matters: Essays in honor of Aaron Wildavsky*. West View Press.

Esmer, Y. (2002a). At the ballot box: Determinants of voting behavior. In S. Sayari & Y. Esmer (Eds.), *Politics, parties and elections in Turkey* (pp. 91–114). Lynne Rienner.

Esmer, Y. (2002b). Is there an Islamic civilization? *Comparative Sociology, 1*(3–4), 265–298.

Fukuyama, F. (1995). *Trust: Social virtues and the creation of prosperity*. Free Press.

Galbraith, D., & Shaver, J. H. (2018). *Religion and fertility bibliography*. Retrieved March 24, 2021, from https://www.evolutionarydemographyofreligion.org/wp-content/uploads/2020/01/religion_fertility_bibliography_9.4.18.pdf.

Hacettepe University Institute of Population Studies. (2019). *2018 Turkey Demographic and Health Survey*.

Harrison, L. E., & Huntington, S. P. (Eds.). (2000). *Culture matters: How values shape human progress*. Basic Books.

Hofstede, G. (2001). *Culture's consequences: Comparing values, behavior, institutions and organizations across nations*. Sage Publications.

Inglehart, R. F. (1977). *The silent revolution: Changing values and political styles among western publics*. Princeton University Press.

Inglehart, R. (1997). *Modernization and postmodernization: Cultural, economic, and political change in 43 societies*. Princeton University Press.

Inglehart, R. (2018). *Cultural evolution: People's motivations are changing, and reshaping the world*. Cambridge University Press.

Inglehart, R. F., & Baker, W. (2000). Modernization and cultural change and the persistence of traditional values. *American Sociological Review*, *65*(1), 19–51.

Inglehart, R. F., & Norris, P. (2003). *Rising tide: Gender equality and cultural change around the World*. Cambridge University Press.

Inglehart, R. F., & Welzel, C. (2005). *Modernization, cultural change and democracy: The human development sequence*. Cambridge University Press.

Inkeles, A. (1983). *Exploring individual modernity*. Columbia University Press.

Inkeles, A., & Smith, D. H. (1974). *Becoming modern: Individual change in six developing countries*. Harvard University Press.

Lakomy, M. (2017). The role of values and socioeconomic status in the education-fertility link among men and women. *Vienna Yearbook of Population Research*, *15*, 121–141.

Norris, P., & Inglehart, R. (2002). Islamic culture and democracy: Testing the "Clash of Civilizations" thesis. *Comparative Sociology*, *1*(3–4), 235–264.

Obasohan, P. E. (2015). Religion, ethnicity and contraceptive use among reproductive age women in Nigeria. *International Journal of MCH and AIDS*, *3*(1), 63–73.

Russell, A., & Thompson, M. S. (2000). Introduction: Contraception across cultures. In A. Russell, M. S. Thompson & E. J. Sobo (Eds.), *Contraception across cultures* (pp. 1–23). Routledge.

Schnabel, L. (2021). Secularism and fertility worldwide. *Socius: Sociological Research for a Dynamic World*, *7*, 1–18.

Schwartz, S. H. (1996). Value priorities and behavior: Applying of theory of integrated values systems. In C. Seligman, J. M. Olson & M. P. Zanna (Eds.), *The psychology of values: The Ontario Symposium, Volume 8* (pp. 1–24). Erlbaum.

Schwartz, S. (2006). A Theory of cultural value orientations: Explication and applications. *Comparative Sociology*, *5*(2–3), 137–182.

Srikanthan, A., & Reid, R. L. (2008). Religious and cultural influences on contraception. *Journal of Obstetrics and Gynaecology Canada. 30*(2), 129–137.

Thornton, A. (2005). *Reading history sideways: The fallacy and enduring impact of the developmental paradigm on family life.* University of Chicago Press.

Thornton, A., Dorius, S. F., & Swindle, J. (2015). Developmental idealism: The cultural foundations of world development programs. *Social Development. 1*(2), 277–320.

Timur, S. (1972). *Türkiye'de aile yapısı.* Hacettepe Üniversitesi Yayınları.

Van de Kaa, D. J. (2001). Postmodern family preferences: From changing value orientation to new behavior. *Population and Development Review*, *27*, 290–331.

Welzel, C. (2010). How selfish are self-expression values? A civicness test. *Journal of Cross Cultural Psychology*, *41*(2), 152–174.

RAHIME SÜLEYMANOĞLU-KÜRÜM

3 Politics of Family Planning in Turkey: Ideological Polarization and Demographic Policies

Abstract: This chapter focuses on the politics of reproductive health and family planning in Turkey and its interaction with population policies. Special attention is paid to the political polarization and politicization of reproductive health policies which, basically, emerged from the ideologies of the governing parties, religious values, and the dichotomy between conservatism and liberalism. Government programs and party manifestos are inspected as partial evidence of the sharp ideological/political polarization in the country. The findings underscore that biopolitical interventions in the life and reproductive health of women reflect path dependency since the 19th century Ottoman Empire and its strategies to expand the population. Even though different population policies have been followed, both in the pro-natalist (pre-1960 and post-2000) and anti-natalist periods (1960–2000), biopolitical measures have focused on controlling women's reproductive rights, with two main types of justification: religiosity and protecting the family.

Keywords: Pro-life, pro-choice, biopolitics, political polarization, population policy in Turkey, pro-natalist policies, anti-natalist policies.

1 Introduction

Population (in size and quality) is perceived to be an important determinant of the economic and political development of societies, constituting a country's active labor force (Coale & Hoover, 2015). As women are widely defined by their reproductive roles, population policies directly involve government intervention in reproductive rights and the autonomy of women. However, development is not a unidimensional issue and cannot be measured solely by looking at economic indicators or quantitative measures, as critics such as Amartya Sen (1999) argue. The most popular indicator of development, gross national income (GNI) per capita, measures development solely in economic terms and ignores other indicators of development, such as health security and living a healthy life or a life with dignity. Population planning policies often lead to the politicization of women's rights and autonomy to control their bodies; such issues become significant in public debates, and the politics surrounding them are increasingly polarized with the involvement of a diverse range of actors (see de Wilde, 2011).

The government's exercise of power and its regulation of life, death, body and sexuality are referred to as "biopolitics", and such regulatory measures touch upon issues of family, widely accepted images and roles of manhood and womanhood. As Deveaux (1994) points out, governments exercise power over fetal protection, issuing laws and new reproductive and genetic technologies that affect women's reproductive rights and autonomy to control their bodies. Debates revolve around whether abortion should be legal or criminalized, encouraged or discouraged, and what determines the population policies of a given state revolves around two types of arguments, which Eric Swank refers to as pro-life and pro-choice groups. The former, according to Swank, approaches the issue of abortion from the perspective of morality, citing religious elements to argue in favor of protecting the life of the fetus, women's health, and familial and traditional values (see also Merola & McGlone, 2011). The pro-choice group, comprised of feminists empowered by second-wave feminism after the 1960s, argues that restrictions on abortions erase women's autonomy over their sexual practices and reproductive decisions (Swank, 2021).

This analysis, conducted at the intersection of population and reproductive policies, triggers (also in Turkey) significant politicization among pro-life and pro-choice arguments. Pro-life arguments are in line with neoconservative ideology, which positions female subjectivity at the center of the government's regulation of individuals and the population and shapes reproduction, sexuality and family policies. Governments enact pro-life policymaking with reference to religion in general but also based on a specific interpretation of religion that excludes and denies the legitimacy of alternative lifestyles and demands (Altunok, 2016). Instead, they focus on the family as a moral and legitimate site of sexuality and assign women the primary responsibility for motherhood. Neoconservatism rejects liberal arguments such as the rights-based claims of individuals – pro-choice arguments – and the plurality of lifestyles, opinions and choices as well as moral perspectives (Altunok, 2016).

This study sets the ground for the empirical analysis to be presented in the subsequent chapters of the volume. It focuses on the politics of reproduction and family planning policies in Turkey and their intersection with population policies. It particularly looks at the political polarization and politicization of reproductive health changes depending on the ideologies of the governing parties, religious values, and the balance between conservatism and liberalism. This chapter relies on primary and secondary data sources. Primary sources are government program[1] and party programs[2] dating back to the establishment of the modern Turkish Republic in 1923, based on keyword searches (women, family, abortion, family planning, population). While the discussions on government programs and their acceptance do not make specific references to the reproductive rights of women, they do display particular perceptions of women and their bodies as political sites for the development of policies in Turkey. The position of women is debated with reference either to women's rights and the process of modernization in Turkey or to development policies. The chapter maps the changes and evolution in the perception of women and the cyclical approach toward women's rights in general and reproductive rights, in particular, through a longitudinal analysis of the post-1923 period.

The chapter starts with key debates on reproductive policies, abortion rights and the feminization of poverty utilizing secondary literature. It then continues with an analysis of population policies of modern Turkey, starting with the pre-1960 period when pro-natal policies were enforced; these policies were replaced by anti-natal policies from the 1960s to early 2000s and then gradually returned to pro-natal policies. After presenting this background, this paper engages in a comparative study of the respective periods and summarizes the ideological polarization in Turkish politics with regard to reproductive rights.

2 Reproductive Policies, Abortion Rights and the Feminization of Poverty

The debates around reproductive policies touch upon three key academic discussions in the literature that I will focus on in this section: (i) religiosity and women's autonomy; (ii) feminization of poverty; and (iii) sexual contract. These debates, however, are interrelated and cannot be discussed without reference to one another. Reproductive rights are often politicized, triggering significant polarization of domestic politics and society. Abortion opponents and pro-life groups seek to discourage abortion by referring to claims such as women's health or religious arguments that equate abortion with murder. States pursuing population expansion policies (so-called pro-natal policies) tend to support measures that limit or even criminalize abortion. However, attempts at criminalization or other measures to discourage abortion trigger further demands to protect women's rights and autonomy over their bodies and significantly impact women's health and poverty, which are the core arguments raised by pro-choice groups, mostly comprised of liberal and left-wing governments. Therefore, the debates between legalization and criminalization of abortion as well as the informal norms and practices that encourage or discourse abortion are most intense in societies marked by deep societal cleavages between (neo)conservatism and liberalism, as well as religiosity.

Studies have shown that highly religious people tend to favor eliminating abortion (Begun & Walls, 2015). For instance, in Nicaragua, the conservative government in power in the early 1990s, as well as the viewpoints of the Catholic church, disseminated a discourse equating all contraceptive methods to abortion, which had a strong impact (Garfield & Glend, 1992). In Muslim societies, the decision to procreate is largely shaped by traditional, familial and religious pressures, and the lower status of women hinders their use of contraceptives (Omran, 2012). In their comparative analysis of "religious and cultural influences on contraception", Srikanthan and Reid (2008) demonstrated that family planning is permitted in Islam as neither family nor marriage is considered an obligatory duty, and contraception is allowed as families have the obligation to ensure the rights of children, i.e., education. Even though some Islamic fundamentalists interpret any form of contraception as a violation of God's will, there are permissible contraceptive methods, such as coitus interruptus, which is recommended in cases of economic inadequacy and health risks, and other modern and lawful methods as long as they are reversible, temporary, and do not lead to abortion (Poston, 2005). Irreversible sterilization methods are not permitted (Hasna, 2003). However, this relatively liberal approach to contraception is hardly transferrable to abortion, which is considered a serious crime equivalent to murder according to Muslim belief. Emergency contraception is also not approved of but is permissible in exceptional circumstances, such as a risk of maternal mortality, a deformed or nonviable fetus, rape and economic indicators.

The conservative and religious ideology of governments and medical professionals usually claims to protect women's health as a justification for their refusal to provide access to legal abortion rather than granting this right and decision to women themselves (Shepherd & Turner, 2018). Kimball and Wissner's (2015) research shows a strong correlation between higher religiosity scores and higher infant mortality rates, while lower abortion rates are associated with voting conservatively and greater income inequality, which has a significant impact on women's health outcomes. While these studies did not make a link between their analysis and the growing literature on the "feminization of poverty" (Peterson, 1987; McLanahan & Kelly, 2006), they reach parallel conclusions, suggesting that women's life chances and capacities are limited by patriarchal norms and state apparatuses that, although they should provide citizens with health security, these services are narrowly interpreted by male authorities who dominate governments and parliaments. The link between these ideologies and clandestine, unsafe abortions must be emphasized, as women are often blamed for becoming pregnant, even though they cannot afford contraception; their choice is to either have to procreate or abort the fetus.

The criminalization of abortion, therefore, does not eliminate abortion but rather drives women to clandestine, unsafe and illegal abortions, together placing further impediments on women's health and exacerbating poverty. Criminalization or other forms of restriction not only reinforce inequalities between men and women but also create and reinstate new vulnerabilities, as women from relatively marginalized racial and ethnic backgrounds or women with limited economic and social capital are disproportionately influenced and further locked into poverty. This was the case in Brazil following the penalization of abortion, which pushed women from marginalized racial, ethnic and socioeconomic backgrounds into greater poverty who were forced to seek clandestine abortions without medical supervision, risking their lives and reinforcing gender and social inequalities (de Almeida Teles, 2006; Cisne et al., 2018). These studies clearly demonstrate that the criminalization of abortion reinforces the feminization of poverty, particularly for women from disadvantaged groups. The correlation between abortion and poverty is also confirmed in Oberman's (2018) study, which has shown that poor women have more abortions than wealthy women because they are more vulnerable to unplanned pregnancy due to lack of access to safe contraceptive methods. In addition to the factors that lead disadvantaged women to seek abortions, the high costs of motherhood often result in lifelong poverty, poor health and mortality for offspring and mothers.

There seem to be two paradoxical arguments with regard to the link between abortion and the feminization of poverty. On the one hand, the right to abortion is argued to empower women by paving the way for them to obtain education and access to career opportunities and thus improve their socioeconomic status. These studies from the so-called pro-choice group focus on women's right to reproductive autonomy, which is the most favored argument in feminist debates as the most obvious solution to the problem of the feminization of poverty (Bandarage, 1998). In contrast, Thomas Strathan's (2014) research, based on a review of 26 studies, revealed that women who have had abortions are more likely to engage in drug and alcohol use to overcome the negative feelings associated with the abortion; they are also more likely to become pregnant again and undergo repeated abortions with a wide range of psychological influences and health problems, making them more likely to need public assistance. While this study is important for underlining access to abortion as not leading to economic prosperity or social well-being, it does not take into consideration the pre-existing poverty of women, which entraps women in the difficult choice of abortion while also triggering further health problems because of the choice of abortion method. Moreover, the author seems to implicitly claim that governments should have the authority to limit access to abortion because of the adverse consequences with no mention of the government's responsibility for eliminating the underlying causes of women's poverty, which encourages them to seek abortion and public assistance in the first place.

Women's reproductive autonomy is hindered not only by government interventions but also by the patriarchal norms and limited education of couples in general and women's education in particular, as well as the husband's desire for more children and the sex preference for the next child (Saleem & Pasha, 2008). In line with the pro-choice groups' arguments, abortion can be an insufficient solution to tackle women's poverty, arguing that criminalizing abortion or limiting women's reproductive autonomy is problematic from a human rights and feminist perspective. We should also account for the welfare state system. The following interventions from Rothman are important and illustrative of the aforementioned debates:

> They [women] are the victims of a social system that fails to take collective responsibility for the needs of its members and leaves individual women to make impossible choices. We are spared collective responsibility because we individualize the problem. We make it the woman's own. She "chooses," and so we owe her nothing. (Rothman, 1986, p. 189)

Arguments raised by pro-life groups or anti-abortion supporters imply that women are selfish and keen on terminating their pregnancies without addressing the underlying causes of poverty. They are encouraged to be self-sacrificing and to allow any kind of manipulation of their bodies. This is because neoconservatism ascribes the central locus of women's lives as being the family (Elomäki & Kantola, 2018). Women, especially marginalized women, are not asked for their consent. Even if consent is demanded, it is often done so by the most privileged women, not the marginalized women who are the most vulnerable. This body politics on abortion is a form of "sexual contract" that men impose on women. Pateman (1988) argues that civil society is created through a patriarchal social order that draws on a "sexual contract" between men and women. In this postpatriarchal and contractual society, men extend civil freedom, which has always been a masculine right, in exchange for establishing a political right over women to create a patriarchy through employment, marriage, prostitution and surrogacy. These contracts emphasize the cultural constructions of womanhood and exclude them from participating in political life by providing men with a disguised legitimacy to govern women's bodies, decisions and lives. In such a fraternal and contractual civil society, abortion policies are indeed perfect tools for men to regulate new forms of access to women's bodies.

3 Population Policies of Modern Turkey and the Ideological Polarization Over Women's Bodies

This section analyzes the population planning and reproductive policies in Turkey and follows the periodization offered by Baştürk (2020) as the choice of population policies overlapped with the evolution of reproductive policies in Turkey. Turkey followed pro-natalist policies until the 1960s, encouraging population expansion and increasing birth rates by framing abortion as a crime, replaced by anti-natalist policies from the 1960s to 2000s aimed at controlling the population. The final subsection addresses the post-2000 period, which marked a gradual return to pro-natalist policies with the declaration of the "at least three children" discourse. The following three subsections analyze how different governments governed reproductive policies with a specific focus on the impact of liberal and neoconservative ideology.

3.1 Pre-1960s: Pro-Natalist Population Policies

Turkey implemented pro-natalist policies until the 1960s, which were supported by social, economic and legal measures to encourage population expansion and increasing growth rates. The initial biopolitics measures, therefore, did not assume the discourse of the right of the fetus to life or the reproductive autonomy of women but rather solely focused on increasing the population to meet the necessary labor force needs of the young republic's agricultural and industrial sectors (see Akşit, 2010). Up until the 1960s, there was a path dependency of the measures implemented in the 19th century of the Ottoman Empire, marking the beginning of government intervention in the area of women's bodies (i.e., opening of public hospitals, compulsory health checks for sex workers) (Miller, 2007). This was enacted through the prohibition of the use of contraception pills in 1838 (justified on religious grounds and interpreted as disobedience of divine will), administrative sanctions on abortion and its eventual criminalization in 1859 (Erkmen, 2020). As criminalization did not prevent women from resorting to abortion, the religious-based claims of the pro-life group were disseminated more strongly, such as defining the termination of a pregnancy as a devilish crime according to the readings of the Koran to discourage women from seeking an abortion while at the same time providing women with incentives to procreate, including a salary and childcare benefits (Erkmen, 2020). In 1926, the Turkish government adopted the Italian Penal Code, which covered abortion as part of "crimes against an individual". It penalized abortion without exception, although there were penalty reductions for men who facilitated a woman aborting because of rape. As such, patriarchal norms and biopolitics interventions have taken women's reproductive autonomy away from them (see Ertem, 2011, p. 52).

The debates in government programs during this period made strong references to the need to follow comprehensive population policies as a reflection of the power of the state. A closer biopolitics reading of the government programs at the time reflects a clear paradox. On the one hand, women's empowerment was prioritized in line with the liberal ideology. For instance, during the single-party government of the Republican People's Party (CHP), the Ali Fethi Bey government in 1923 promised to pay equal value for the education of boys and girls.[3] On the other hand, given the need to increase the population, the same CHP ideology, following the paths of Atatürk's modernization paradigm, associated women with family, as illustrated by the issuance of a series of laws (i.e., 1930 the General Hygiene Law) that encouraged women to reproduce (i.e., rewards and medals to women having six or more children, prohibiting the sale of abortion tools) (Akın & Aykut, 2011) and adding special courses to the education curriculum for girls to prepare them for familial responsibilities.

In reviving the legal measures that fall into pro-natal policies, it is important to underline the celibacy tax debates that emerged in the early republican period. This bill was first voiced by Hamdi Bey (an MP from Canik) in 1921, requiring unmarried men over the age of 20 to pay a tax. While this proposal was not accepted at the time, it remained on the agenda, with a more comprehensive proposal submitted by another MP (Salih Efendi) 4 months later and again by Yozgad Deputy Sırrı Bey during the 1929 Depression (Özer, 2013). These proposals were rejected, but the design of a comprehensive population policy was central and openly stated in the presentation of the government program by Prime Minister Celal Bayar in 1937, with additional measures such as the establishment of village midwife schools for safe births in villages.[4] Further measures to increase fertility included reducing the age of marriage with a change to the Civil Code in 1938 (from 18 to 17 for men and from 17 to 15 for women), criminalizing abortion and birth control, tax exemptions, reward systems for families with many children, and incentives to young people to marry (see Bozbeyoğlu, 2011; Baştürk, 2020).

While the measures during this period reflect a path dependency since the 19th century, with abortion being placed under the heading of offenses against the integrity of race, the debates over population policies in the deliberations over government programs started to reveal alternative and more conservative voices within the party. This is evident in the statement of an MP, Sırrı Içöz, who underlined the necessity of interfering with the uniforms of female civil servants by pointing out the potential drawbacks they may cause.[5] On the one hand, women were assigned full work responsibility in the private sphere; therefore, they should be educated to become good mothers and professionals with equal rights. On the other hand, they were also attributed full responsibility for upholding the "honor" of society, reflecting a conservative ideology and greater religiosity. For instance, Refik Şevket Ince, an MP from Manisa district, who later became a founding member of the more conservative Democrat Party (came to power in 1950), delivered a statement underlining his hope that women would dress in a way that did not damage the youth (implying their morality) and invited women to work with dignity.[6] Following the shift to the multiparty system in 1946, such voices became more vocal and visible in government programs. The most illustrative statements were delivered by Sinan Tekelioğlu during the deliberations of Şemsettin Günaltay government, who criticized the number of women bureaucrats for being too high, pointing out the potential complications this would cause regarding marriage. Inviting the government to take action in this direction, Tekelioğlu continued as follows:

> It should be the top priority of the state and the government to seek remedies to marry them. We are well aware that none of the women working in the directorate could get married. It is also a responsibility for the government to find remedies for this. Because there will come a time when the population in the country will decrease completely and there will be no marriages, the country will go toward a disaster. For this, it should be the first duty of the Şemsettin Günaltay Government to find a solution.[7]

Importantly, Sinan Tekelioğlu, an MP from Adana, was also involved in the formation of a more conservatively oriented Democrat Party, such as Refik Şevket Ince mentioned above. These debates have already signaled an emerging opposition, which is more religiously oriented and has a more conservative approach toward the role of women in society. This opposition sponsored extensive debates on women's bodies, clothes and looks, and linked the debates to honor issues. In fact, when the Democrat Party came to power in 1950, during the presentation of the government program, Suad Hayri Ürgüblü, a CHP MP from Kayseri, asked the government how it would handle the population issue; he pointed out that population growth alone does not lead to the development of nations, stressing the importance of investing in the quality of the population and improving the value of the labor force, its skills and morality.[8] However, even in the second term of the Democrat Party, during the presentation of the government program in 1954, the promise to take measures to increase the population was retained,[9] although it became clear that population growth led to unsustainable growth.

3.2 1960s to 2000s: Anti-Natalist Policies

After the second half of the 1950s, Turkey's demographic structure started to be transformed, with increasing fertility reaching a 28.5 % population growth rate, making Turkey one of the countries with the highest rates of population growth (Hoşgör & Tansel, 2010). Along with increasing life expectancy, welfare systems such as education, health, housing and social security came under pressure to sustain the growing population, requiring a shift to anti-natalist policies (Baştürk, 2020). The first concrete achievement in this regard was the establishment of the State Planning Organization in 1960, which installed a new population policy in cooperation with the Ministry of Health and Social Assistance. The need to handle population growth and development is also underlined in the First Five-Year Development Plan and the Law on Population Planning adopted in 1965, which allowed the sale, import and application of birth control methods. However, the emerging discourse in government programs made barely any reference to women's right to have autonomy over their bodies or reproductive rights. It is also important to note that religiosity and conservative attitudes grew since the Democrat Party came into power, removed from power in 1960 (by a coup d'etat), although various parties continued to capture its voter base (Bulut, 2009). The Justice Party (AP), led by Süleyman Demirel, incorporated conservative elements into its liberal ideology, resulting in another entrapment of women in familial roles, as revealed in the following statement in the presentation of his government program in 1969 and repeated in its election manifesto in 1973[10]:

> It is among our goals to facilitate the daily life of women in accordance with the great and sacred position of the Turkish family and to allow them to fulfill their duties at home in peace. The goal of our development and thus our developing economy is to provide prosperity in the country. Health, social and cultural services addressing housewives will be increased. These will be provided cheaply and easily.[11]

Family planning emerged for the first time in the presentation of the same government program with a question asked by an MP from the opposition party CHP (Sadi Koçaş), asking the government's view on the application of the law on family planning and birth control and adding that it is essential to start with the East rather than the West due to the former's lack of access to these opportunities.[12] In contrast, the chair of the Nationalist Action Party, Alparslan Türkeş, also drew attention to the birth control policy and stated the following:

> Birth control is not a measure to be applied for Turkey. If most of the population in our country is compared with other countries, it will be seen that there is no fear of population growth in our country yet. The development of our country is possible with the

> exploitation and utilization of our wealth. It is not the right way to consider population control as a remedy.[13]

Although the new population policy adopted in 1960 marked the official shift to an anti-natalist policy, abortion remained criminalized but allowed under some exceptional circumstances, e.g., when the health of the mother and fetus were at risk. Nevertheless, the abortion debate became increasingly politicized and was brought into parliamentary deliberations by liberal parties, revealing maternal deaths due to illegal abortion and the inability to reduce the population growth to the desired level (Aba et al., 2016). As Erkmen (2020) showed, in the 1970s, such debates intensified, with stronger calls for the liberalization of abortion leading to a number of bills offered by political party representatives from liberal and left-leaning parties such as the CHP (by Celal Kargılı and four others) and Justice Party (Nazım Baş) as well as Senator Nermin Abadan Unat, but they were all rejected by conservative parties in the parliament.

The analysis of government programs reveals greater politicization around population planning policies, with all short-lived governments presenting family planning policies with justifications for improved women's and children's health, as well as the associated problems of urbanization, unemployment and limited resources to sustain the growing population. During this period, CHP ideology pursued a greater agenda for women's liberation, with extensive deliberations on resisting religiosity that limited women's lives.[14] Despite the extensive politicization around the issue of reproduction, family planning and abortion in the Turkish Parliament, abortion was not liberalized until 1983. Erkmen (2020) illustrates that it was only after the 1980 coup that a bill and an amendment to the Turkish Penal Code was offered, pointing out the already dysfunctional abortion ban and touching upon justifications for its decriminalization such as women's health and the feminization of poverty. Evidence was provided to illustrate how the illegality of abortion preserved access for women from the middle or upper classes while further marginalizing women from lower socio-economic backgrounds, depriving them from the right to terminate a pregnancy, and leading to greater poverty, health risks and even death due to unsafe abortion practices.

Abortion was eventually liberalized in 1983 (with law no. 2827 on Population Planning) with setting out the conditions under which pregnancy can be terminated and the uterus can be evacuated, limiting further sterilization and contraction surgery beyond the cases stipulated by this law. As such, the state established a monopoly in deciding how to use the bodies and lives of women rather than granting them decision-making autonomy. The most debated issue, according to Erkmen (2020), was the requirement of husbands' permission for the termination of pregnancy, reflecting a patriarchal mindset while leaving many uncertainties about who controls women's bodies.

Such a discourse is strongly related to the emerging neoliberal and neoconservative ideology, which manifested itself most strongly in the discourse of the Motherland Party (ANAP) that came to power in 1983 and was reelected and/or formed governments in 1987 and 1989. The ANAP associated women primarily with the family, defining her as the most important element of society and critical for economic development. This stance is also retained by subsequent governments, including the True Path Party (DYP) under the leadership of Süleyman Demirel, which came to power in 1991 and established a Ministry of Women, Family and Child Protection, promising to eliminate obstacles for the establishment of youth and female branches of political parties, insurance to housewives, and women-specific programs.[15] It can be argued that the role attributed to women expanded beyond the family (investing in their education) by the True Path Party (DYP) government under the leadership of Tansu Çiller, who became Turkey's first female Prime Minister in 1995 even though she had been criticized for paying little attention to the family.[16] In fact, when assuming power after Çiller, ANAP's neoconservative ideology was revived under Mesut Yılmaz's leadership (a coalition of the ANAP and DYP) with a stronger association of women with the family. This is indicated by Mesut Yılmaz's three-month-long government from March to June 1996, which authored the phrase, the "*woman is the most authoritative, directing, nurturing, unifying and protective element of the family position*". This view was identical to how Prime Minister Necmettin Erbakan, from the conservative and religiously oriented Welfare Party that served in a coalition with DYP from 1996 to 1997, approached the role of women in society:

> Our woman is the most effective director and nurturer of the family, which is the smallest and basic institution of society, and is an individual who has equal responsibilities with her husband in creating the happiness and well-being of the family. Efforts will be focused on eliminating the negative conditions affecting the place of Turkish women in society. In particular, necessary measures will be carried out to increase the education, health, employment and social status of women. The protection and development of the family, which is the cornerstone of society, will be essential.[17]

The following phrase from the party program of the Nationalist Work Party (Milliyetçi Çalışma Partisi-MSP) is largely illustrative of the political ideology of conservative parties in Turkish politics in the 1980s:

> We strongly reject attacks on the family and its social functions under the guise of feminism. However, we believe that it is necessary to defend women and their rights and

> protect women as a respected creature together with their men. We do not agree with population growth being the only factor preventing economic development. We believe that the productive character of the population should be mobilized. … We reject an understanding of abortion as a tool for population planning because abortion is a result of not having access to contraception and inability to make the necessary planning. We will change the current practice of exposing women to permanent abortion by pushing protection to the second plan.[18]

In sum, by the end of the 1950s, government representatives realized that the rapid expansion of the population would cause economic and social problems, triggering a shift to anti-natalist policies aimed at controlling population growth, consisting of a series of measures and laws that eventually legalized abortion in 1983. During this period, the presentation of government programs was highly politicized around the issue of population growth and limited resources, both by the governing and opposition parties. However, we observe continuity in terms of targeting the bodies of women, justified by the lives and health of women and infants and the role of the women in the family. Only with the coming into power of a new government in 1997, under the leadership of Prime Minister Bülent Ecevit (Democratic Left Party-DSP), was women's familial role abandoned and replaced by a more concrete gender equality agenda in line with its liberal ideology, in which women's empowerment was equated with Turkey's modernity and democracy and women's education was prioritized.[19]

3.3 Post-2000s: Revival of Pro-Natalist Policies

Liberal ideology and women's empowerment, largely economic, were retained until at least 2006. However, when the Justice and Development Party (AKP) came into power in 2002, there was a revival of the politicization around the issues of abortion and population decline, as had been the case before the 1960s. AKP's pro-natalist policy was clear from a 2003 proposed bill to restrict abortions after the 10th week, which was annulled due to reactions from the media, women's NGOs and medical associations at the time (Acar & Altunok, 2013). Despite the government's neoliberal and neoconservative ideology, there has not an official, but rather a gradual, de facto shift to pro-natalist policies with implicit statements in development programs underlining the need to prioritize Turkey's demographic potential with no further roadmap of policies and strategies to be adopted (Baştürk, 2020).

In contrast to the AKP's neoconservative pro-life arguments, there have been pro-choice arguments coming from the Socialist Democracy Party program since 2003, underlining the party's vision of opposing discrimination against women in all legal, economic, political and social fields with explicit references to the slogans "our body is ours", "only the woman has the right to decide on the prevention or termination of pregnancy", and "the government should never intervene in women's choice to give birth to children or not". The program also underlined that women should be free to choose the method of abortion or contraception, both of which should be free, and private centers established for the provision of services.[20] This argument was also widespread among feminist groups and women NGOs fighting for women's liberation and emancipation. However, this was against the ideology of the ruling AKP party, which underscored the philosophical and political core of its declared "conservative ideology" was to keep the family healthy and together.[21] Erdoğan's speech closely resembled Özal's neoconservative ideology, as it presented a discourse on women making up half of society and "raising healthy generations". Hence, women have been treated as being instrumental to maintaining effective population policy. This approach has been criticized by the CHP opposition party for viewing women as merely a device for the continuation of the population; they invited the government to treat women as the foundation of society instead.[22] Another MP from the AKP, Ömer Çelik, reacted to these criticisms with the following statement:

> The statement whether a woman is treated as a device for the reproduction of the generation is disrespected for the institution of maternity under the cover of respect for women. A woman is respectful for us both as an individual and as a mother. Women's individual and motherhood missions are not alternatives or conflictual areas with each other.[23]

This statement reflects the AKP's balancing of its neoconservative approach with its liberal standing, which has been argued as being instrumental for AKP to gain legitimate ground for winning liberal and secularist votes to consolidate its power, although they were adopted as "tick box" legislative exercises (Cin & Süleymanğlu-Kürüm, 2021). Especially since its second electoral victory in 2007, the AKP associated women more strongly with family and its elites established rigid expectations on how women should behave in public. As it consolidated its power, the party gradually replaced its discourse on women's rights with the protection of the family. Such a shift of focus was clearly observable in the 2007 government program, which indicated:

> The family is the cornerstone of society. All social values build on the solidity of this foundation. Together with all our institutions that bear social responsibility for the strengthening of our social fabric and the safety of our future generations, we have to give importance to the family institution and the protection of family values more than ever.[24]

Since 2011, an anti-women or pro-natal discourse has become much more visible and consistent with neoconservative ideology. First, the Ministry of State Responsible for Women and Family was replaced by the Ministry of Family and Social Affairs in 2011. Subsequently, the prioritization of the family paved the way for a series of measures to grant care services to women (Acar & Altunok, 2013), the introduction of "flexible" employment packages and privileging maternity leave and parental follow-ups over contraception and abortion, and dissemination of anti-scientific information on women's bodies to women by clerics (Dayı & Karakaya, 2018). Subsequently, in 2012, Erdoğan went as far as to declare abortion and Cesarean sections (because it reduces the maximum number of births) as murder, hindering Turkey's economic growth potential (Korkut & Eslen-Ziya, 2016). He equated abortion to the Uludere event, which resulted in the killing of 34 Kurdish citizens and interpreted such practices as an attack on Turkey's dynamic population growth (Altınok, 2016). Even more extreme is the declaration by Recep Akdağ, the Minister of Health, arguing that women should not abort a baby even in cases of rape (Dayı & Karakaya, 2018). Such a discursive construction of pro-life arguments and accusing women of acting selfishly by ending their pregnancies at the expense of the life of an innocent fetus has put pressure on medical providers, leading to a decline in abortions and use of contraception, especially intrauterine devices, in public hospitals (Dayı & Karakaya, 2018). Hence, there has been a de facto ban on abortions in state hospitals, forcing women to seek unsafe, clandestine abortions (Altunok, 2016; Erkmen, 2020).

Upon Erdoğan's election as President, the new Prime Minister Ahmet Davutoğlu made a stronger emphasis on women's welfare and adopted the Istanbul Convention (Council of Europe Convention on the Elimination of Domestic Violence against Women in 2011). In the presentations of the government programs (64th and 65th government), concepts such as "preservation of family" and "dynamic population" are used together with references to women's individual and social development.[25] Additionally, in line with its neoliberal ideology, the discourse was centered on promoting women's education to encourage women's entrepreneurship and employment, particularly the "reconciliation of work and family life".[26] These assertions reveal that the government's perception of women's empowerment does not entail women's ability to make strategic life choices that she previously lacked (Kaaber, 1999). It prioritizes women's economic welfare and development, rather than treating women as ethical subjects and taking women's agency and dignity as priorities.

While the guiding ideology was clearly neoconservatism, a wide range of justifications were provided by the AKP government, such as population decline and aging, the transformation of the public health systems, the right to life of a fetus, and so-called pro-life arguments. The population argument was put forward in the Tenth Five-Year Development Program, drafted in 2013 and announced in 2015, explicitly pointing out the need to develop effective policies to increase fertility and sustain the dynamic characteristics of the population complementing the "at least three children" policy and discourse that the then Prime Minister, now President, Erdoğan, had adopted in 2009 (Eryurt et al., 2013; Baştürk, 2020; Dayı & Karakaya, 2018). Therefore, even though there has not been any official change in policy, pro-natal policies are argued to have been revived at the discursive and informal levels (see Oktay, 2014; Dayı & Karakaya, 2018). That is, women were again equated with the family and assigned the primary responsibility of giving birth.

4 Ideological Polarization in Turkish Politics on Reproductive Rights: Comparative Analysis

Government intervention in life and women's reproductive choice has been present throughout the period under analysis, as both pro-natalist and anti-natalist periods have treated women's uterus as a policy issue of the state in shaping their population policies. This is because women's claim for autonomy over their reproductive choices contradicts the state's "right over life" (Altunok, 2016). Nevertheless, justifications for these positions have changed among the periods. Religiosity-based arguments and conservativism emerged as driving factors for the type of government intervention in the politics of women's bodies and life. When these findings are evaluated with the evolution of Turkish politics, ideological polarization is clearly manifest. As Kalaycıoğlu (2007) noted, the Democrat Party (1950 and 1954), Justice Party (in 1965 and 1969), Motherland Party (1983 and 1987) and Justice and Development Party (2002) were milestones of democratic politics in Turkey. Importantly, each of these dates has seen a shift toward conservative/neoconservative ideas around biopolitics.

During the pre-1960 period, biopolitical justifications relied on familial structure and religiosity, while the main concern was insufficient population and the need to expand the population base to ensure the economic development of the young republic. Throughout this period, particularly after 1950, religious-based and pro-life arguments were disseminated to women to discourage them from demanding the right to abortion. In the second period, from 1960 to the 2000s, a growing population, along with urbanization and rising unemployment, led to measures to gradually loosen restrictions on abortion and eventually to its legalization. While greater emphasis had been given to women's education during this period, the main motivation was not to give birth to more children but rather to support women in becoming good mothers and to raise future generations with greater visibility for pro-choice arguments, particularly related to the achievements and mobilization of second-wave feminism. However, it is wise to argue that abortion politics in both periods were shaped by economic concerns and nationalist policies as well as development-oriented regulations through controlling life rather than any concern for human rights or for providing women with autonomy over their bodies (Akşit, 2010; Erkmen, 2020).

Since the coming into power of the Motherland Party in 1983, the subsequent True Path Party (DYP) as well as other parties positioned in the right-of-center, adopted a neoconservatist ideology that combined "political conservatism and economic liberalism" (Kalaycıoğlu, 2007). As these parties have been struggling to obtain peripheral votes, neoconservatism became their defining ideology, and their approach to women's rights and empowerment followed the same ideology. In the third period that started in the early 2000s, there was neither an official change of policy nor any amendment to the abortion law, but there was a de facto discursive shift toward pro-natalist policies that promoted pro-life arguments limiting women's access to abortion and birth control. Unlike the previous two periods, there has been an increase in the visibility of neoliberal measures and conservative politics, triggering nationalist and sexist reactions (see also Dayı & Karakaya, 2018; Erkmen, 2020). In fact, several scholars have noted that, similar to Margaret Thatcher and Ronald Reagan, the AKP favored neoliberal politics while relying on conservative values concerning religion and family – combined liberalism and conservatism – in what is known as neoconservatism or the rise of right-wing politics that center on anti-women policies and policies that assign women to familial roles (Gambetti, 2009; Dayı & Karakaya, 2018).

Such an ideological position serves as an evident disruption of the achievements of feminists in Turkey and of their dissemination and eventual consolidation of pro-choice arguments. With the emerging de facto pro-natalist policies, particularly after 2008, the debate once again turned to the strategy of controlling and regulating women's reproductive rights instead of diverting attention to women's social problems or policies such as parental leave, fiscal incentives, family benefits or tax reductions as alternative strategies. Rather, the focus was on coercive measures to constrain contraception, ignoring feminist arguments that pro-natal policies dictate a sociality that privileges the patriarchal order and traps women in their "traditional roles" while perpetuating their secondary position in society (Akşit, 2010). Erdoğan's reaction to abortion, especially his equation of abortion to Uludere, is argued as being a clear manifestation of his government's neoconservative ideology, controlling female subjectivities through biopolitics (Altunok, 2016). Even though this attitude has triggered many reactions from medical associations and women NGOs, their pro-choice and rights-based arguments have been consistently ignored. Women became the central focus, defined in traditional and patriarchal forms as discussed in the previous section. The AKP also benefitted from the neoliberal turn and the flourishing of civil society organizations in the early 1990s, most of which defined themselves as religious and conservative and have been fighting against headscarf bans (Altunok, 2016).

5 Conclusion

The population policies of the modern Turkish Republic carry the legacies of the weakening of the Ottoman Empire and the remnants of many years of struggle, the loss of the Muslim population, the loss of veterans from wars (i.e., Balkan Wars, First World War and the War on Independence) and the loss of women and children caused by diseases. The size and quality of the population shaped the choice of pro-natalist or anti-natalist policies, implemented through the intervention of biopolitics into life and reproductive health and legitimized with religiosity arguments or population structures.

This chapter focused on the politics of reproductive health and family planning in Turkey and its interaction with population policies. In particular, it looked at the political polarization and politicization of reproductive health at the intersection of family planning and population policies that emerged from the ideologies of the governing parties, religious values, and the dichotomy between conservatism and liberalism, using evidence from government and party programs as well as secondary literature. The findings underscore that biopolitical interventions in the life and reproductive health of women reflect path dependency since the 19th century Ottoman Empire and its strategies to expand the population. Even though different population policies have been followed, both in the pro-natalist (pre-1960 and post-2000) and anti-natalist periods (1960–2000), biopolitical measures have focused on controlling women's reproductive rights, with two main types of justification: religiosity and protecting the family.

None of the periods have demonstrated dominance by pro-choice arguments by governing parties, apart from the feminist movement. The representation of pro-choice arguments by political parties remained marginal and dispersed by political parties that had not managed to form a government by capturing sufficient votes to secure an electoral victory. In other words, even though there have been significant manifestations of both arguments (pro-life and pro-choice) in Turkish society, their representation at the governmental level was rather marginal and mostly limited to the AKP period from 2000 to 2006, during which measures aimed at women's liberation were rather instrumental and largely aimed at gaining a wider spectrum of votes in a polarized Turkish political landscape.

Notes

1. Open Access Link to government programs: https://acikerisim.tbmm.gov.tr/handle/11543/141
2. Open Access Link to government and party programs: http://acikerisim.tbmm.gov.tr
3. Ali Fethi Bey's Speech. TBMM Zabıt Ceridesi Devre 2 Cilt 1 Içtima 14 Sayfa 419–428 5 Eylül 1339 (1923)
4. Celal Bayar (Izmir-Prime Minister), TBMM Zabıt Ceridesi Dönem 5 Cilt 20 Inikad 3 Sayfa 19–42, 08.11.1937.
5. Sırrı Içöz (Yozgad), TBMM Zabit Ceridesi Dönem 8 Cilt 1 Inikat 3 Sayfa 27–71, 14.08.1946.
6. Refik Ince (Manisa) TBMM Zabıt Ceridesi Devre 5 Cilt 29 Inikat 28 Sayfa 214–220, 27.01.1939.
7. Sinan Tekelioğlu (Seyhan) TBMM Tutanak Dergisi Dönem 8 Cilt 15 Birleşim 36 Sayfa 162–206, 24.01.1949.
8. Suad Hayri Ürgüblü (Kayseri), TBMM Tutanak Dergisi Dönem 9 Cilt 1 Birleşim 4 Sayfa 42–92, 31.05.1950.
9. Adnan Menderes (Istanbul-Prime Minister) TBMM Tutanak Dergisi Dönem 10 Cilt 1 Içtima Fevkalade Inikat 3 Sayfa 21–34, 24.05.1954
10. Justice Party Electoral Manifesto (Adalet Partisi Seçim Beyannamesi, 1973) TBMM Kütüphanesi, Yer: 76–187; DEM: 76–320. file:///C:/Users/rahim/Downloads/197600320_1973.pdf, p. 73.
11. Başbakan Süleyman Demirel. TBMM Tutanak Dergisi Devre 3 Cilt 1 Birleşim 4 Sayfa 43–70, 07.11.1969.
12. Sadi Koçaş Cumhuriyet Senatosu Tutanak Dergisi Toplanti Yili 5 Cilt 31 Birleşim 4 Sayfa 44–98 05.11.1965.
13. Alparslan Türkeş, MHP. Millet Meclisi Tutanak Dergisi Devre 3 Cilt 1 Birleşim 4 Sayfa 43–70, 07.11.1969.
14. Ismet Inönü (Malatya-Prime Minister) – Cumhuriyet Senatosu Tutanak Dergisi Toplanti Yili 1 Cilt 4 Birleşim 76, 04.07.1962, pp. 359–411.
15. Süleyman Demirel (DYP-Prime Minister) TBMM Tutanak Dergisi Dönem 19 Cilt 1 Birleşim 7 Sayfa 109–138, 25.11.1991.

16. I. Çiller Hükümeti, 25.06.1993–05.10.1995
17. Necmettin Erbakan. TBMM Tutanak Dergisi Dönem 20 Cilt 7 Birleşim 70 Sayfa 524–539, 03.07.1996.
18. Nationalist Labor Party Program (1988)- Milliyetçi Çalişma Partisi Programi (1988), p. 8. https://acikerisim.tbmm.gov.tr/bitstream/handle/11543/743/199501865-1988.pdf?sequence=1&isAllowed=y
19. I. Çiller Hükümeti, 25.06.1993–05.10.1995
20. Socialist Democracy Party Program (2003) Sosyalist Demokrasi Partisi Program ve Tüzük (2003). https://acikerisim.tbmm.gov.tr/xmlui/handle/11543/898
21. Recep Tayyip Erdoğan (Prime Minister-AKP), TBMM Tutanak Dergisi Dönem 22 Cilt 8 Birleşim 49 Sayfa 118–137, 18.03.2003.
22. Mustafa Özyürek (CHP), TBMM Tutanak Dergisi Dönem 22 Cilt 8 Birleşim 49 Sayfa 118–137, 18.03.2003.
23. Ömer Çelik (AKP). TBMM Tutanak Dergisi Dönem 22 Cilt 8 Birleşim 49 Sayfa 118–137, 18.03.2003.
24. Recep Tayyip Erdoğan (AKP-Prime Minister), TBMM Tutanak Dergisi Dönem 23 Cilt 1 Birleşim 9 Sayfa 131–179, 03.09.2007.
25. 65. Hükümet program, Başbakan Binali Yildirim 24 Mayis 2016 Sali
26. Ahmet Davutoğlu (AKP-Prime Minister), TBMM Tutanak Dergisi, 26. Dönem16. Cilt, 1. Yasama yili, 92. Birleşim, 24 Mayis 2016.

References

Aba, Y. A., Aba, G., Özkan, Ş., & Güzel, Y. (2016). Abortion policies around the world and in Turkey and its reflection on women's health. *International Journal of Human Sciences, 13*(1), 1651–1665.

Acar, F., & Altunok, G. (2013). The "politics of intimate" at the intersection of neo-liberalism and neo-conservatism in contemporary Turkey. *Women's Studies International Forum, 41*, 14–23.

Akın, A., & Aykut, N. B. (2011). Nüfus politikasının oluşturulmasında Türkiye deneyimi. *Sağlık ve Toplum Dergisi. 3.*

Akşit, E. E. (2010). Geç Osmanlı ve Cumhuriyet dönemlerinde nüfus kontrolü yaklaşımları. *Toplum ve Bilim, 118*, 179–197.

Altunok, G. (2016). Neo-conservatism, sovereign power and bio-power: Female subjectivity in contemporary Turkey. *Research and Policy on Turkey, 1*(2), 132–146.

Amélia de Almeida Teles, M., & translated by Bracale-Howard, S. (2006). Women's human rights in Brazil. *Peace Review: A Journal of Social Justice, 18*(4), 485–490.

Bandarage, A. (1998). *Women, population and global crisis: A political-economic analysis*. Zed Books.

Baştürk, Ş. (2020). Türkiye'de nüfus ve demografik yapının dönüşümü. In M. Zencirkıran (Ed.), *Dünden bugüne Türkiye'nin toplumsal yapısı* (pp. 303–338). Dora Yayınları.

Begun, S., & Walls, N. E. (2015). Pedestal or gutter: Exploring ambivalent sexism's relationship with abortion attitudes. *Affilia, 30*(2), 200–215.

Bozbeyoğlu, A. Ç. (2011). Doğurganlık kontrolünde rasyonelliğin sınırları: Türkiye kürtaj ve gebeliği önleyici yöntem kullanımı. *Fe Dergi, 3*(1), 23–37.

Bulut, S. (2009). 27 Mayıs 1960'tan günümüze paylaşılamayan Demokrat Parti mirası. *Süleyman Demirel Üniversitesi Fen-Edebiyat Fakültesi Sosyal Bilimler Dergisi, 2009*(19), 73–90.

Cin, F. M., & Süleymanoğlu-Kürüm, R. (2021). Alternative explanations from feminist theories: Towards a feminist framework for the Europeanisation process. In R. Süleymanoğlu-Kürüm & F. M. Cin (Eds.), *Feminist framing of Europeanisation* (pp. 63–84). Palgrave Macmillan.

Cisne, M., Castro, V. V., & Oliveira, G. M. J. C. D. (2018). Unsafe abortion: A patriarchal and racialized picture of women's poverty. *Revista Katálysis, 21*(3), 452–470.

Coale, A. J., & Hoover, E. M. (2015). *Population growth and economic development*. Princeton University Press.

Dayı, A., & Karakaya, E. (2018). Transforming the gendered regime through reproductive politics: Neoliberal health restructuring, the debt economy and reproductive rights in Turkey. *Les cahiers du CEDREF. Centre d'enseignement, d'études et de recherches pour les études féministes*, (22), 158–192.

Deveaux, M. (1994). Feminism and empowerment: A critical reading of Foucault. *Feminist Studies, 20*(2), 223–247.

De Wilde, P. (2011). No polity for old politics? A framework for analyzing the politicization of European integration. *Journal of European .Integration, 33*(5), 559–575.

Elomäki, A., & Kantola, J. (2018). Theorizing feminist struggles in the triangle of neoliberalism, conservatism, and nationalism. *Social Politics: International Studies in Gender, State & Society, 25*(3), 337–360.

Erkmen, S. (2020). *Türkiye'de kürtaj: AKP ve biyopolitika*. Iletişim Yayınları.

Ertem, E. C. (2011). Anti-abortion policies in late Ottoman Empire and early republican Turkey: Intervention of state on women's body and reproductivity, *Fe Dergi, 3*(1), 46–55.

Eryurt, M. A., Canpolat Beşe, Ş., & Koç, I. (2013). Türkiye'de nüfus ve nüfus politikaları: Öngörüler ve öneriler. *Amme Idaresi Dergisi, 46*(4), 129–156.

Gambetti, Z. (2009). Iktidarın dönüşen çehresi: Neoliberalizm, şiddet ve kurumsal siyasetin tasfiyesi. *Istanbul Üniversitesi Siyasal Bilgiler Fakültesi Dergisi, 40*, 145–166.

Garfield, R. S., & Glen, W. (1992). *Health care in Nicaragua: Primary care under changing regimes*. Oxford University Press.

Hasna, F. (2003). Islam, social traditions and family planning. *Social Policy & Administration, 37*(2), 181–197.

Hoşgör, Ş., & Tansel, A. (2010). *2050'ye doğru nüfusbilim ve yönetim: Eğitim, işgücü, sağlık ve sosyal güvenlik sistemlerine yansımalar*. TÜSIAD. https://tusiad.org/tr/yayinlar/raporlar/item/5187-2050ye-dogru-nufusbilim-ve-yonetim-- gitim--isgucu--saglik-ve-sosyal-guvenlik-sistemlerine-yansimalar

Kabeer, N. (1999). Resources, agency, achievements: Reflections on the measurement of women's empowerment. *Development and Change, 30*(3), 435–464.

Kalaycıoğlu, E. (2007). Politics of conservatism in Turkey. *Turkish Studies, 8*(2), 233–252.

Kimball, R., & Wissner, M. (2015). Religion, poverty, and politics: their impact on women's reproductive health outcomes. *Public Health Nursing, 32*(6), 598–612.

Korkut, U., & Eslen-Ziya, H. (2016). The discursive governance of population politics: the evolution of a pro-birth regime in Turkey. *Social Politics: International Studies in Gender, State & Society, 23*(4), 555–575.

McLanahan, S. S., & Kelly, E. L. (2006). The feminization of poverty. In J. S. Chafetz (Ed.), *Handbook of the sociology of sender* (pp. 127–145). Springer.

Merola, N. A., & McGlone, M. S. (2011). Adversarial infrahumanization in the abortion debate. *Western Journal of Communication, 75*(3), 323–340.

Miller, R. A. (2007). Rights, reproduction, sexuality, and citizenship in the Ottoman Empire and Turkey. *Signs: Journal of Women in Culture and Society, 32*(2), 347–373.

Oberman, M. (2018). Motherhood, abortion, and the medicalization of poverty. *The Journal of Law, Medicine & Ethics, 46*(3), 665–671.

Oktay, E. Y. (2014). Türkiye'de Cumhuriyet'in ilanından günümüze uygulanan nüfus politikaları. *Yalova Sosyal Bilimler Dergisi, 4*(7), 31-53.

Omran, A. R. (Ed.). (2012). *Family planning in the legacy of Islam*. Routledge.

Özer, S. (2013). Cumhuriyet'in ilk yıllarında bekârlık vergisi'ne ilişkin tartışmalar. *Gazi Akademik Bakış, 12*, 173–192.

Pateman, C. (1988). *The sexual contract*. Stanford University Press.

Peterson, J. (1987). The feminization of poverty. *Journal of economic issues, 21* (1), 329-337.

Poston, L. (2005). Islam. In C. Manning & P. Zuckerman (Eds.), *Sex and religion* (pp. 181–197). Wadsworth.

Rothman, B. K. (1986). *The tentative pregnancy: Prenatal diagnosis and the future of motherhood.* Viking.

Saleem, A., & Pasha, G. R. (2008). Women's reproductive autonomy and barriers to contraceptive use in Pakistan. *The European Journal of Contraception & Reproductive Health Care, 13*(1), 83–89.

Sen, A. (1999). *Commodities and capabilities.* Oxford University Press.

Shepherd, L., & Turner, H. D. (2018). The over-medicalization and corrupted medicalization of abortion and its effect on women living in poverty. *The Journal of Law, Medicine & Ethics*, *4*(3), 672–679.

Srikanthan, A., & Reid, R. L. (2008). Religious and cultural influences on contraception. *Journal of Obstetrics and Gynaecology Canada, 30*(2), 129–137.

Strahan, T. W. (2014). *Studies suggesting that induced abortion may increase the feminization of poverty.* Feminism & Nonviolence Studies. http://www.fnsa.org/v1n3/strahan.html

Swank, E. (2021). The gender conservatism of pro-life activists. *Journal of Women, Politics & Policy*, *42*(2), 124–1

Part Two Dimensions of Fertility Behavior: An In-depth Study of a Multi-faceted and Controversial Issue

IQBAL H. SHAH

4 Studying the Impact of a Community-based Family Planning Intervention in Ghana, Pakistan, Tanzania and Turkey: Strengths and Challenges

Abstract: This chapter provides an overview of an innovative project assessing the implementation and impact of a community-based intervention to generate demand for family planning in Ghana, Pakistan, Tanzania and Turkey. The research project was implemented from 2017 to 2020 and was designed to follow a random sample of women from communities selected for the intervention and from the comparative sites where no intervention was planned. Quantitative research methods were used to collect data from women, exit interviews of clients and for surveying health facilities and pharmacies. In-depth interviews were conducted with community stakeholders and health care providers to ascertain community perspectives and insights on family planning and reproductive health. The chapter covers the design of the project, details of implementation, strengths and limitations, and concludes with recommendation for similar efforts in future.

Keywords: Family planning, community-based intervention, contraceptive prevalence, induced abortion, Willows model.

1 Introduction

Contraceptive use, a novelty in the 1960s, rose rapidly in much of the world to become a norm. Contraceptive prevalence – generally measured as the percentage of women of childbearing age (15–49 years) currently married or in union using any contraceptive method – is not available for the period before 1965. However, it was estimated to be above 65 % in the developed world, but only 9 % in developing regions during 1960–1965 (Bongaarts, 1984). Contraceptive prevalence is projected to have reached 71.1 % in the developed and 61.7 % in the developing regions in 2020 (United Nations, 2020). The increase in developing regions has been sustained and – in historical terms, very rapid. However, this global trend masks country and regional variations. The high level of unmet need for family planning also continues to persist in some countries. The progress has been uneven with Sub-Saharan Africa and some countries in South Asia lagging behind.

Family planning interventions were initially introduced to reduce fertility and population growth for sustainable development. However, the pivotal role of contraceptive use in meeting couples' fertility goals and its health benefits for women and children were soon recognized as well as its contribution to expanding female education, labor force participation and empowerment. It is estimated that in 2008, 44 % of maternal deaths were averted by contraception. In addition, 29 % of maternal deaths can be averted each year if unmet need for contraception is fully met (Ahmed et al., 2012).

While unmet need indicates the latent demand for family planning not met by the available services and programs, raising the demand through information and counseling is critical for achieving reproductive goals and improving health and well-being. Much more efforts have been directed to addressing supply-side issues of family planning than to generating demand. Provision of information and services through community-based programs have shown positive results for contraceptive uptake in many settings. Nine of the 11 studies from Ethiopia, China, India, Ghana, Bangladesh, Zambia, Mali, Cameroon and Syria show a positive and statistically significant impact of community-based counseling, education and information programs on contraceptive uptake amongst women aged 15 to 49 (Rupasinghe et al., forthcoming). Further, interventions implemented for longer than 18 months and that adopted a multi-pronged approach were more likely to reduce fertility and increase contraceptive uptake.

This chapter describes an innovative research project that was undertaken to evaluate the impact and implementation of a community-based demand generation program by the Willows International. We first provide a description of the Willows model, followed by the design and implementation of the research project and conclude with key findings, challenges, and recommendations for future studies.

1.1 The Willows Model

Since its launch in 1999 in Izmir, Turkey, the Willows International (formerly named Willows Foundation) model of Community-Based Reproductive Behavior Change (CRBC) has been expanded to millions of women in over 60 sites in Ghana, Pakistan, Tanzania and Turkey. The two main objectives of the Willows model are to inculcate knowledge of reproductive health and instill improved long-lasting reproductive behaviors among underserved groups of women and couples. While keeping the core elements of the Willows model intact across different countries where Willows International works and over time within each country, the model has been adapted to local conditions and needs. In general, Willows management, in consultation with the Ministries of Health, selects a region for the implementation. Once the region is selected, underserved areas are identified in consultation with regional health and other administrative authorities (provincial directorate of the Ministry of Health in case of Turkey). The identified project areas are generally inhabited by low-income and less educated migrants from rural areas. Services in such areas are generally available, but underutilized by women. Once the project area has been selected, women community workers (Field Educators) are recruited and a project office is established with a coordinator, two assistants to manage data entry, one supervisor per 10 Field Educators, and Field Educators (FEs). FEs are selected from amongst those living in the project community, aged 18 years or older, with at least 5 years of schooling and good communication skills. They are trained for 3 weeks and only those who successfully complete the training are recruited. FEs generally do not receive salary, but are compensated for expenses related to transportation and meals. Their monthly compensation is about one-third of that paid to a fresh graduate of midwifery.

The intensive FE training program focuses on communication skills and includes, among other topics, (a) importance of healthcare during pregnancy and signs and symptom to watch out for during and after delivery; (b) effective contraceptive methods for preventing unintended pregnancy; (c) benefits and side effects of different contraceptive methods, and the choice of appropriate and acceptable method; and (d) where, how, and at what price are reproductive health services available in the area. The focus of training is primarily on uptake and continuation of modern contraceptive methods. In addition to the initial training program, weekly meetings are organized in the project office throughout the program's implementation and at the request of FEs, where information on the implementation and challenges encountered are discussed and solutions are found. Further, the Willows trainers provide a 40-hour refresher training to review all topics within the first 3 months following basic training and after the household assessment. Additional refresher courses are organized, as needed, depending on the length of the project implementation.

Once training is successfully completed, each FE is assigned to cover a designated number of clients, about 1,000 married women of reproductive age (15–49 years) in Turkey but varies from country to country depending on each country's specific situation. For example, in Ghana all sexually active women, irrespective of marital status, were reached by FEs. Each woman is visited at least 4–5 times on average. Women who meet the Willows' criteria for priority attention are placed in priority groups and are visited more often while there may be some women who receive one or even no visit after the baseline is completed.

Willows priority groups are determined based on a woman's contraceptive needs identified by the responses she provided to the baseline questionnaire. Willows management information system (MIS) allows women to move among priority and non-priority groups as their status and needs change during the project implementation allowing FEs to visit women who are in need of Willows services.

FEs provide information to women, their husbands, and, when requested, to single youths living in the same household. The purpose of the visit is to impart reproductive health knowledge to make informed choices. Those who seek a service are referred to a local health care facility of their choice. Women, or their husbands, who have been referred to a health care facility are revisited after the referral. Access to both public and private health care facilities is supported by the project through an agreement with the Ministry of Health and by establishing a close collaboration with private providers in the project area.

In the first 3 months of the project, FEs visit households to conduct a household survey using a client information form (CIF) both to describe essential demographic and reproductive background characteristics and to identify the particular needs of women. In this preliminary visit, data are collected on women's age, education, pregnancy history, contraceptive practice, and knowledge of reproductive health. The needs in terms of pregnancy prevention, pregnancy health care, and general health care are assessed from the information provided in CIF. Then, a follow-up visitation card is created for each married (or sexually active in Ghana and Tanzania) woman of reproductive age (15–49 years) in the household. The next step is to determine the priority class into which each woman is assigned according to her needs. After the completion of the household assessment, the FEs receive a brief refresher training and then they initiate the home visits. During the course of project implementation, the previous steps are repeated for newcomers to the area and for any women who were not assessed previously. During home visits, counseling on modern contraceptive methods takes priority over other services.

Which women should be visited each week is determined electronically by the special software developed for the Willows International and the client cards belonging to these women are placed in the FE's boxes by the supervisors. Additionally, supervisors and the field office manager may manually add a small number of client cards after a weekly review of the cards. Each FE has a certain number of client cards assigned per week, including back-up cards. This number varies from country to country. For example, in Turkey about 125–150 cards are placed in FE boxes weekly and each FE is expected to carry out 15 to 20 home visits per day. The number of client cards placed in FE boxes and the number of women visited each week are smaller in other countries. Priority is given for a follow-up visit to women who are pregnant, who have recently had a delivery or abortion, those not using contraception, and those who are lactating. Second priority is given to newlyweds, engaged couples, and users of traditional methods.

Following each visit, the information provided and the situation identified are recorded on the computer to monitor a woman's reproductive health care needs and status. Electronic monitoring and evaluation is among the many unique and strong features of the Willows model. FEs report any changes in the status of women they follow and enter on the computer. These reports are individually checked and verified in the field by field coordinator before submission to the project office. Data are then transferred to the Willows office in Istanbul where such data are analyzed to monitor the progress of the project and performance of FEs and project offices. The system also allows the identification of needs and timely feedback to project areas for improving implementation. In addition, a manual monitoring and evaluation system classify all women by their reproductive needs for follow-up. For example, pregnant women will be followed up and referred to facilities for antenatal care while women wanting no more children but not using a method will be referred for contraceptive services. The manual "box" system permits follow up of users of modern methods, users of traditional methods and non-users.

Recent adopters of modern methods are closely followed for the first 6 months to address any issues or concerns with the use of the method. Women who are dissatisfied with the method are visited every month for counseling and for facilitating switching to another method for continued protection against unintended pregnancy. FEs describe the experience of women who were referred and visited a health facility. Those referred but who have not visited the health facilities are encouraged to visit and some are accompanied by FEs.

The following groups of women are generally visited once every 4 to 6 weeks: (1) Women who do not use a traditional method effectively; and (2) Women who are not using any method, although they do not desire to have more children.

Every pregnant woman is visited in her early, mid and late pregnancy. Those women, who are in their last months of pregnancy, but have never been visited, are given priority. Every nursing mother is expected to be visited at least once during the first 42 days after delivery, to encourage uptake of effective contraception, and to find out if she is experiencing any health problems. Breast feeding is promoted mainly for the nutritional needs of the new-born and for child health than for its contribution to contraceptive protection.

The following groups of women are visited once every 6 months:

(1) Women who use traditional methods effectively,
(2) Satisfied users of a modern method for at least 6 months,
(3) Women aged over 35, and
(4) Women who want to have a child and have given birth more than 2 years ago.

In Turkey and Pakistan, women who are never married, divorced, or widowed are not given a "priority" with regard to reproductive health services, but information on reproductive health is provided, if requested. Services provided to husbands and adolescents, mostly on weekends, are also recorded on the women's survey cards.

The FEs are not expected to provide contraceptive supplies, but do provide methods, when requested, to the first time user, and a pack of iron supplements to pregnant women. They also distribute printed educational materials. Services provided by the Willows include, but not limited to, (1) the provision of information and education to women; (2) referrals for service; and (3) follow up of the method adopted and referral service used.

Following a study in 2001, collaboration with health institutions in project sites was strengthened, especially to improve communication skills of FEs and providers, improving management capacity of health facilities and the infrastructure to provide counseling in privacy. Willows International provides technical training for improving patient-provider communication and may support contraceptive supply, especially in project areas that experience shortage of contraceptive commodities. After meetings in each province in Turkey where project was launched, Willows Foundation (International) started to award "Most-Friendly Health Institution" award, every 3 months, to recognize the improvement in quality of service provided and to promote good collaboration between the project staff and service providers. Workshops on interpersonal communication and on reproductive health were organized in several provinces for service providers.

Support from the community leaders are sought through frequent meetings and consultations. They are also consulted for identifying FEs. The type of community leaders approached differ by country – religious leaders in Turkey and Pakistan and village chiefs or elders in Ghana – and so does the degree of support and collaboration.

Extensive and regular supervisory checks are routinely carried out and feedback is provided to facility coordinators and to FEs. The basic structure and phases of the Willows model have remained largely intact since 1999. The "core" of the model requires that all eligible women in the project areas are identified using the baseline data and classified into priority groups with the highest priority given to women who do not want to have another child or have the next child after 2 years, but not using any method. Each FE is required to visit women identified for a timely and customized service. FEs are required to follow up referrals diligently and those women who were referred but did not go must be visited and reasons noted.

The implementation of the model in sites in Ghana and Pakistan and, more recently, in Tanzania, offered an opportunity to consider if the model is replicable outside Turkey. While the core elements of the model have remained largely intact, the fidelity by which the core elements have been implemented over time and across countries was a question of scientific and programmatic interest. Other differences between Turkey and other countries are also noteworthy. While the focus of the intervention in Turkey and Pakistan is on married women, all sexually active women in project sites are covered in Ghana and Tanzania. Also, FEs include both men and women in Ghana and Tanzania, while only female FEs are deployed in Turkey and Pakistan. In addition, the length of the intervention varied across countries and sites within a country. Another noticeable change is in the lengthening of the project duration from an average of 18 months previously in Turkey to 2 years or longer in recent project sites.

Information and data about the experience and outcomes of implementing the Willows model have now been accumulated from project sites varying in degree of application, duration of implementation and from different demographic, sociocultural and service contexts. It was, therefore, appropriate to consider the impact and implementation of Willows model to inform future programming.

2 Research Project: Implementation and Impact Evaluation of the Willows' Reproductive Health Programs in Ghana, Pakistan, Tanzania and Turkey

At the invitation of the long-standing Sponsor of Willows International, Harvard T.H. Chan School of Public Health (HSPH) developed the project research proposal. The development of proposal was facilitated by a pre-proposal grant by the Sponsor to visit all four countries for in-depth discussions with Willows country staff as well as with potential research project partners and for meetings with the Sponsor. In order to better inform the development of the proposal and to decide on research study design and procedures, we also conducted a systematic review of evidence on community-based interventions to improve contraceptive uptake. The review was also necessary to learn the experience in implementing relevant community-based interventions and the gaps identified by studies evaluating their impact.

The project proposal was approved in 2017 and the project was launched in a meeting involving all country project staff, Willows International Staff, Harvard project team, and the representatives of the Sponsoring agency. The four country project partner organizations included: Regional Institute of Population Studies, Accra, Ghana; Aga Khan University, Karachi, Pakistan; Kilimanjaro Christian Medical University College, Moshi, Tanzania; and Bahçeşehir University, Istanbul, Turkey. Dr. Ayaga Bawah was the principal investigator for Ghana, Dr. Sajid Soofi for Pakistan, Dr. Sia Msuya for Tanzania and Dr. Yılmaz Esmer for Turkey.

The overall goal of the project was to provide data and analysis that can be used to inform future programmatic decision-making, both for the Sponsor as well as for the Willows International. Using a quasi-experimental, prospective design involving Willows program and matched comparison sites, the evaluation aimed to measure the impact of the Willows' model in creating behavior change among women of reproductive age with regard to uptake and continued use of modern contraceptives in Ghana, Pakistan, Tanzania, and Turkey. More specifically, the evaluation was to measure the effects of the Willows program on contraceptive prevalence (CPR) over time, with particular focus on modern methods of contraception (mCPR), from baseline to 2 years or more after the end of the intervention period. In addition, the evaluation was to investigate how the impact of the intervention varied across different communities and between specific subgroups of women by education, wealth quintile, age, parity, and contraceptive use at baseline. Through a detailed process evaluation, the project also aimed to document how the Willows model was implemented in each country, paying particular attention to documenting how the Willows model was adapted to meet specific cultural and contextual needs of each community. Two additional objectives included the assessment of the effectiveness of the Willows model in increasing women's knowledge of, access to, and use of locally-based reproductive healthcare services and to produce estimates of the cost per client served and the cost per induced new user and continued user of a modern conceptive method that can be linked to exposure to the Willows program. The project activities to meet these objectives were divided into two components.

2.1 Component 1: Prospective Process and Impact Evaluation

To measure the impact of the Willows model and sustained behavior change, a robust prospective design was developed covering baseline data and longitudinal follow-up of women in a representative sample of households in program and matched comparison sites to determine changes in use of modern methods that can be attributed to the Willows model. To select a representative sample of households, we first identified and mapped a geographical area from within the area covered by the Willows program. We identified a similar area in terms of population size, number of households and ethnic/language composition in the comparison area that was geographically not adjacent to the intervention area. This was then followed by a complete household listing in both the selected program and comparison areas. From the list, we planned to randomly select about 2,500 households in order to achieve the sample of 2,000 eligible women for the interview. Each sample household was approached to identify women eligible for interview.

There were four intervention sites, pre-selected by the Willows International, for the prospective studies based on planned interventions by Willows in 2017 and 2018, one each in Ghana, Pakistan, Tanzania, and Turkey (Tab. 4.1). For each proposed program site, we selected, in discussion with the Willows country and headquarter staff, a matched comparison area with similar characteristics. The selection of matching area was guided by the data available on: (a) the number of women 15–49; (b) whether the community is slated to be a Willows program site in the future; (c) socio-economic characteristics such as income and educational level of the community; (d) cultural characteristics such as dominant ethnicity, language or religion; (e) whether or not the community was receiving migrants and, if yes, from where, by geographic sub-units. In addition, we reviewed maps identifying proposed intervention and control areas to ensure they were not adjacent so as to minimize spillover effects. While comparison areas were similar to the program areas, they were not randomized and so there could be systematic differences between program and comparison women. In order to control for this, during the analysis phase, we used a statistical matching procedure of coarsened exact matching (Iacus et. al, 2012), matching each woman in the treatment area with a woman in the control area with very similar baseline characteristics such as age, education, work status, parity, marital status, and current use of modern contraceptive methods.

In addition to the baseline and follow-up surveys of eligible women, this component of project proposal included: (i) a facility survey, (ii) analysis of the Willows MIS data, (iii) in-depth qualitative interviews with women and FEs, (iv) in-depth documentation and process evaluation in each program area, and (vi) collection of cost data, including program costs per site, and where possible costs per component (e.g., household visits, salaries of staff, community outreach activities), overhead costs, and service utilization rates. To this list, pharmacy surveys and exit interviews of clients were added during the implementation. However, in 2019, the Sponsor decided to conclude the project without the planned follow-up surveys at the end of the intervention and later. In-depth qualitative interviews were conducted with community stakeholders and not with women and FEs as originally proposed. Thus, all of the analyses of data were based on the baseline cross-sectional surveys of women, facility and pharmacy surveys, exit interviews and the analysis on Willows MIS data. Table 4.1 shows the data collected for Component 1 and Tab. 4.2 shows the number of in-depth interviews conducted with stakeholders in Willows program sites. Overall, 16,587 women were interviewed, 104 facilities and 1,346 pharmacies were surveyed and 1,590 exit interviews were conducted with clients in the four countries. In addition, 76 qualitative in-depth interviews were conducted with stakeholders including health providers and community leaders.

2.2 Component 2: Retrospective Implementation and Effectiveness Assessment

Component 2 of the project covered the sites that had recently completed a Willows program. Originally, three program and matching comparison areas in three out of the four countries: Ghana, Pakistan, and Turkey were identified. However, the Sponsor decided to drop Turkey. We carried out a one-time cross-sectional household survey around 18–24 months after the end of the Willows program in each site. The survey covered 4,236 women in program sites and 4,191 women in the matched comparison sites in Ghana and Pakistan (Tab. 4.3). Using this cross-sectional survey of woman, we were also able to undertake the validation and analysis of the Willows MIS data. This component of the study was intended to produce results more rapidly than the prospective component. The drawback of the retrospective approach is that it required that we collect information based on women's recall rather than contemporaneously. The prospective longitudinal study set out in component 1 above is comprised of a more robust design, the retrospective study provided results is a much timelier manner and at a very low cost to inform future programming.

The retrospective surveys were, by their nature, different from the longitudinal study questionnaires. They asked questions about past as well as current activities. A key element of the retrospective study was assessing women's contraceptive use over the 3 to 5 years prior to the survey covering the Willows baseline and endline and project's post-program follow up period. These data were crucial both for estimating impact of the program and for validating the Willows MIS data. While in the retrospective component, the calendar data provided baseline (prior to Willows intervention) information on contraceptive use, such data in the prospective component provided a unique opportunity of validation. The calendar uses event histories for women by a series of questions about the timing of pregnancies and births followed by probing woman's contraceptive use between pregnancies to create a complete month by month record of contraceptive practice. This approach is used for histories of 5–6 years prior to survey by the Demographic and Health Surveys (DHS) and is widely accepted as a valid method (Bradley et al., 2015). In retrospective component, only surveys of eligible women were undertaken and no additional data were collected for facilities or for in-depth interviews.

3 Key Findings and Program Implications

We also undertook an analysis of Willows MIS data by matching with data collected in retrospective surveys in Ghana and Pakistan and estimated cost per new user. The original project proposal was approved for 6 years, including surveys at the end of intervention and follow up surveys at 1 and 2 years later. However, the Sponsor decided to end the project before the planned period and, therefore, the endline and post-program surveys, and process evaluation were not realized. A number of publications utilized the project data for in-depth analysis of high priority topics (see Tab. 4.4).

The findings from surveys of women, facilities, and pharmacies supplemented by exit interviews and key informant interviews (KIIs) revealed a nascent yet complex mosaic of fertility regulation in the four countries. While knowledge of contraceptives is nearly universal, important differences exist across countries with regard to method choice and general availability of contraceptives and of specific methods. The levels and rate of increase in modern contraceptive prevalence (mCPR), main reason for discontinuing a method, and the most prevalent reproductive status at 3 months after discontinuation may indicate underlying differences in fertility regulation trajectories by country. In Ghana and Tanzania, the percentage of women who are pregnant at 3 months post-discontinuation are close to the percentage experiencing method failure or discontinuing because of the desire to become pregnant. However, in Pakistan and Turkey, many more women are pregnant at 3 months since discontinuation – 39.4 % and 49.5 %, respectively – than women who experience method failure or who discontinue because of the desire to become pregnant (19.7 % in Pakistan and 9.3 % in Turkey). Neither the lack of availability of methods, nor the quality of service seem to explain these differences. Ambivalence toward family planning was noted in the narratives of KIIs in Pakistan and, to some extent, Turkey. Additional in-depth studies are needed to fully understand the dynamics and trajectories of contraceptive use in the four countries; however, demand generation and information dissemination interventions are justified in these settings. Other program implications and recommendations are as follows.

4 Program Implications

Taken together, the study findings indicate the following recommendations:

- Counseling and information provision should be tailored to women's particular situation, needs, and reproductive preferences. This requires client-focused counseling rather than standardized counseling covering all possible methods and topics.
- In contexts where attitudes toward family planning continue to be ambivalent among certain groups, for example in Pakistan, health benefits of birth spacing for infant, child and maternal survival, and family wellbeing, must be incorporated into counseling and information interventions.
- While a focus on modern methods, and especially on long-acting methods, is well justified for longer-term protection against unintended pregnancy, women who use traditional methods need to be supported and informed on how to use those methods consistently and correctly. We note that countries with high overall contraceptive prevalence (Pakistan and Turkey) show significant reliance on traditional methods, but with high failure rates.
- There is a need to provide correct information about family planning and contraceptive methods to dispel myths and misperceptions regarding side effects, method safety, and efficacy.
- The high prevalence rates coupled with high discontinuation rates offset gains made by increasing contraceptive uptake. There is an urgent need for programs and interventions to prioritize continuation of use by providing information on potential side effects and how to manage them. The programs also need to assist women in switching to a method that meets their needs and preferences in a timely manner.
- The switching in methods calls for programs to ensure regular supply and stocks of different methods. Timely switching to a method of choice prevents unintended pregnancy and strengthens rights-based family planning.
- Demand generation interventions coupled with supply of contraceptive methods and/or effective and timely referral is potentially more effective than generating demand only.

- Addressing gaps in choice of methods that are available and improving the quality of service can potentially increase the uptake and prolong the use of a method.
- The narratives from key informant interviews highlight the importance of engaging community stakeholders (including women's groups, pharmacists, and religious leaders) and service providers, and involving men to improve program effectiveness.
- The variety of contraceptive use patterns and contexts call for interventions to be tailored to local service and cultural settings.

5 Implications for the Willows Model

The key implications and recommendations are as follows:

1. The extent to which Willows program is able to reach eligible women in the community influences the uptake of contraceptive use and, therefore, prevalence of modern contraceptives (mCPR). The coverage of community registration and enrolment of clients must be strengthened and complete for the program to achieve its intended objectives and outcomes. We found the coverage to be woefully inadequate in Ghana and Pakistan where retrospectives studies were conducted.
2. Those women and couples who moved into the program area need to be registered and followed-up. The Willows MIS data show limited numbers of women registered after the initial baseline registration.
3. The long period of registration of clients and even longer period from registration to first counseling visit can lead to some women having unintended pregnancies before the first home-based counseling visit by the Willows FE. The counseling visits by FEs could be launched in parallel with registration. The gap between registration and first contact must be reduced to the minimum to promptly address the unmet need for contraception and prevent unintended pregnancies.
4. Given the high discontinuation rates and little timely switching to another effective method, low priority accorded to users of modern methods at baseline registration need to be revised. Women using short-term spacing methods, whether traditional or modern, need to be visited more frequently and assisted with changing methods, if desired, to improve continuation of contraceptive protection.
5. Multiple visits are needed to generate contraceptive uptake among non-users. The odds of use increase rapidly as the number of visits grows, for example, from five in Pakistan and seven in Ghana.

6 Strengths and Limitations

The research project was exceptional in its rigorous design and implementation. Team members diligently followed best practices for research, including obtaining ethical approvals, informed consent, pilot-testing instruments, household listing, representative sampling, interviewing, data quality and analysis. Household surveys of women were complemented by surveys of facilities, pharmacies, drug stores to map out the provision of reproductive health services and exit interviews were conducted with clients to ascertain their satisfaction with the service received. Contextual information was obtained by interviewing key informants who were knowledgeable and influential in the community on matters related to sexual and reproductive health. Therefore, the project was able to cover the key dimensions of demand for and supply of fertility regulation services.

The use of electronic tablets with built-in skip patterns and quality checks allowed team members to collect and manage high quality data. Electronic tablets facilitated the teams in implementing a robust quality assurance protocol with built-in, automated checks to ensure consistency, identify erroneous entries in real time, and minimized missing data. Survey instruments underwent several rounds of internal testing by research team and further piloting locally. Based on findings from research team review and pilot tests, team members made improvements to the survey instruments before implementation. The instruments were translated from English to local languages and back-translated and trained enumerators collected data under the supervision of senior researchers.

The data collected permitted pursuing innovative research ideas and application of analytical techniques; for example, applying geo-spatial analysis of contraceptive method use and the location of health facilities. Another strength of the project is the potential for linking different datasets, such as facility surveys, exit interviews and women's surveys. This enabled the project team to examine the distance-quality trade-off in women's choice of family planning provider by linking women's data with facility data. In addition, the measurement of quality of services was facilitated by linking facility data with exit interviews.

Facility and pharmacy surveys covered all facilities identified by available records, supplemented by visits to the study areas. In addition, facilities indicated by women in the cross-sectional surveys (Component 1) were included for data collection. Exit interviews collected no personal identifying information and were conducted in private places to ensure confidentiality and privacy. Several rounds of revisions of interview guide, pre-testing and training in interviewing preceded the interviews.

The project has some limitations. Similar to other surveys, we cannot rule out the potential of recall errors, especially in calendar data and for women with complex reproductive histories. The training in collecting information for the calendar was extensive. In addition, the length of calendar was relatively shorter (31 months before the survey) than in Demographic and Health Surveys (60 months) and can be assumed to have fewer recall errors.

As in other surveys, women in all countries may have underreported the induced abortion experience. In Ghana, the level of underreporting appears less than in the other three countries. Reporting errors cannot be ruled out for facility and pharmacy surveys. Exit interviews with clients and in-depth interviews with key informants can be affected by "courtesy" bias.

7 Challenges and Recommendations

A critical challenge for the study design was that each Willows program is carried out in a single cohesive large site. This made it impossible to undertake a randomized controlled trial with randomization either at the woman level or cluster randomization with numerous small clusters without fundamentally changing the nature of the model. The program sites are pre-selected. We, therefore, had to rely on the next best approach of finding a comparable site that matched with the program area. While comparison areas were similar to the program areas they were not randomized and so there could be systematic differences between program and comparison women. In order to control for this, during the analysis phase, we used a statistical matching procedure of coarsened exact matching, matching each woman in the program area with a woman in the comparison area with very similar baseline characteristics such as age, education, work status, parity, marital status, and current use of modern contraceptive methods.

The selection of the comparison sites was not straightforward despite the objective criteria used. The requirement that intervention and comparison areas were geographically distinct to avoid any spillover effects was difficult to ensure. Indeed, the sites initially selected in all four countries had to be changed and, in Ghana, the change in comparison site took place after interviews with over 50 % of eligible women were completed in the initially selected site.

The future studies evaluating a program or intervention should preferably use a randomized controlled approach. This approach automatically provides balance between the program (treatment) and comparison (control) groups with the two differing only in the treatment except by chance.

Another formidable challenge was to match the data from retrospective surveys with Willows MIS data. Given that MIS data were to have a complete coverage of all eligible women in the program area and interviews were conducted with a sample of women from the same area, it was anticipated that most of women residing in the area throughout the period from the start of the Willows program to our survey would be found in both datasets. The exact matches were, surprisingly, few – 16 % in Ghana and 5 % in Pakistan. This low level of matching of survey and MIS data made the detailed analysis unwarranted.

The timing to initiate baseline registration by the Willows International was close to the baseline project surveys. This required coordination of activities and adjustments in scheduling interviews. However, data in all sites were successfully collected before the start of Willows baseline registration.

Perhaps the most serious challenge was the truncation of project by the Sponsor canceling the planned and surveys at the end of the Willows program and process evaluation. The project was, therefore, unable to realize its full potential and meet all of the approved objectives it set out to address. The decision by the Sponsor to drop Turkey from the retrospective component was another violation of the approved project protocol.

Our experience offer two main recommendations for future evaluation studies. First, when possible, the evaluation studies should consider a randomized controlled design. Second, the project should ensure full implementation and adherence to the approved protocol and plans. The project funding agreement should, therefore, include a binding clause for the funder and the grant recipient to implement all approved project activities.

In conclusion and despite the various challenges it faced, the project generated some very important findings, which Willows can use for developing and improving future programming. The cross-sectional data from the baseline, facility survey, pharmacy survey, and exit interviews, provided rich insights into the current state of reproductive health, particularly on contraceptive use, in poor urban settings of Ghana, Pakistan, Tanzania, and Turkey. Country Willows teams and other stakeholders (e.g. policy makers, researchers, health officials, etc.) can use these data as a baseline for future research, implementation of sexual and reproductive health programs, prioritizing underserved groups, and improving continuation of contraceptive use and timely switching of methods. The capacity strengthened by designing and implementing the project helped build skills for data collection, qualitative and quantitative data analysis, and manuscript preparation, skills that the team will use far beyond the conclusion of the project.

Tab. 4.1: Data collected as part of component 1: Prospective process and impact evaluation

	Ghana	**Pakistan**	**Tanzania**	**Turkey**	**Total**
Program site	Osu Klottey, La, Teshie, Nungua; Accra.	Jamshed Town; Karachi.	Sokoni, Daraja, and Sinon; Arusha.	Bağcılar; Istanbul.	
Comparison site	La Nkwantanang, Agbogba, and Old Ashongma, Madina; Accra.	Yousuf Goth; Karachi.	Akeri and Usariver; Meru.	Küçükçekmece; Istanbul.	
Number of women final sample (both areas)	4,180	4,245	3,938	4,224	**16,587**
Number of women (program area)	2,178	2,080	1,956	2,112	**8,326**
Number of women (comparison area)	2,002	2,165	1,982	2,112	**8,261**
Facilities surveyed: program area	27	22	29	26	**104**
Facilities surveyed: comparison area	34	8	10	9	**61**
Number of pharmacies surveyed	354	358	508	126	**1,346**
Number of exit interviews completed: program area	453	142	125	241	**961**
Number of exit interviews completed: comparison area	458	46	55	70	**629**

Tab. 4.2: Key informant interviews (KIIs) conducted in component 1: Prospective process and impact evaluation

	Ghana	Pakistan	Tanzania	Turkey	Overall
Number of stakeholders interviewed	24	22	14	16	76
Number of service providers interviewed	11	10	7	8	36
Number of community stakeholders interviewed	13	12	7	8	40

Tab. 4.3: Data collected in the retrospective household survey, Ghana and Pakistan

	Ghana	Pakistan	Overall
Program site	[Osu Klottey, La, Teshie, Nungua; Accra]	[Korangi Town, Karachi]	
Comparison site	[La Nkwantanang, Agbogba, and Old Ashongma, Madina; Accra]	[P.I.B. Colony and Dalmia, Karachi]	
Women interviewed in Program site	2,168	2,068	**4,236**
Women interviewed in Comparison site	2,062	2,129	**4,191**

Tab. 4.4: List of project publications[1]

Bawah A. A., Sato R., Asuming P., Henry E. G., Agula C., Agyei-Asabere C., Canning D, & Shah I. (2021). Contraceptive method use, discontinuation and failure rates among women aged 15–49 years: evidence from selected low income settings in Kumasi, Ghana. *Contraception and Reproductive Medicine*, 6:9. https://doi.org/10.1186/s40834-021-00151-y.

Elewonibi B., Amour C., Gleason S., Msuya S., Canning D., & Shah I. (2020). Estimating the lifetime incidence of induced abortion and understanding abortion practices in a Northeastern Tanzania community through a household survey. *Contraception*, https://doi.org/10.1016/j.contraception.2020.10.013.

Elewonibi B., Sato R., Manongi R., Msuya S., Shah I., & Canning D. (2020). The distance-quality trade-off in women's choice of family planning provider in North Eastern Tanzania. *BMJ Global Health*, 2020;5:e002149. doi:10.1136/ bmjgh-2019-002149.

Hackett K., Henry E., Hussain I., Khan M., Feroz K., Kaur N., Sato R., Soofi S., Canning, & Shah, I. (2020). Impact of home-based family planning counselling and referral on modern contraceptive use in Karachi, Pakistan: a retrospective, cross-sectional matched control study. *BMJ Open*, 2020;10:e039835. doi:10.1136/bmjopen-2020-039835.

Tab. 4.4: Continued

Hackett K., Huber-Krum S., Francis J. M., Senderowicz L., Pearson E., Siril H., Ulenga N., & Shah I. (2020). Evaluating the implementation of an intervention to improve postpartum contraception in Tanzania: A qualitative study of provider and client perspectives. *Global Health: Science and Practice,* June 2020, 8(2):270–289; https://doi.org/10.9745/GHSP-D-19-00365.

Henry E. G., Hackett K. M., Bawah A., Asuming P. O., Agula C., Canning D., & Shah I. (2020). The impact of a personalized, community-based counselling and referral program on modern contraceptive use in urban Ghana: a retrospective evaluation. *Health Policy and Planning,* doi: https://doi.org/10.1093/heapol/czaa082.

Huber-Krum S., Hackett K., Kaur N., Nausheen S., Soofi S., Canning D., & Shah I. (2020). An application of the list experiment to estimate abortion prevalence in Karachi, Pakistan. *International Perspectives on Sexual and Reproductive Health,* 46, Supplement No. 1, Focus on Abortion: 13–24.

Huber-Krum S., Karadon D., Kurutas S., Rohr J., Baykal S., Okcuoglu B. A, Esmer Y., Canning D., & Shah I. (2020). Estimating abortion prevalence and understanding perspectives of community leaders and providers: Results from a mixed-method study in Istanbul, Turkey. *Women's Health,* 16:1–13.

Khan M.B., Nausheen S., Hussain I., Hackett K., Zehra K., Feroze K., Canning D., Shah I., & Bashir S.S. (2021). Conducting household surveys on reproductive health in urban settings: lessons from Karachi, Pakistan. *BMC Medical Research Methodology,* 21:38. https://doi.org/10.1186/s12874-021-01216-x.

Kurutas S., Sato R., Huber-Krum S., Baykal S. S., Rohr J., Karadon D., Kaur N., Okcuoğlu B. A., Esmer Y., Canning D., & Shah I. (2021). Contraceptive discontinuation and switching in urban Istanbul region in Turkey. *International Journal of Gynecology and Obstetrics.* https://doi.org/10.1002/ijgo.13577.

Sato R., Rohr J., Huber S., Esmer Y., Okçuoğlu B. A., Karadon D., Shah I., & Canning D. (2021). Effect of distance to health facilities and access to contraceptive services among urban Turkish women. *The European Journal of Contraception & Reproductive Health Care.* https://doi.org/10.1080/13625187.2021.1906412.

Sato R., Elewonibi B., Msuya S., Manongi R., Canning D., & Shah I. (2020). Why do women discontinue contraception and what are the post-discontinuation outcomes? Evidence from the Arusha Region, Tanzania. *Sexual and Reproductive Health Matters,* 28:1, 1723321, DOI: 10.1080/26410397.2020.1723321.

Özçelik EA., Rohr J., Hackett K., Shah I., & Canning D. (2020). applying inverse probability weighting to measure contraceptive prevalence using data from a community-based reproductive health intervention in Pakistan, *International Perspectives on Sexual and Reproductive Health,* 46:21–33, doi: https://doi.org/10.1363/46e8520.

Note

1. Editor's note: The following articles were published after the list compiled by the chapter author:

   Karadon, D., Esmer, Y., Okcuoglu, B. A., Kurutas, S., Baykal, S. S., Huber-Krum, S., Canning, D., & Shah, I. (2021). Understanding family planning decision-making: Perspectives of providers and community stakeholders from Istanbul, Turkey. *BMC Women's Health*, *21*(1), 357. https://doi.org/10.1186/s12905-021-01490-3

   Huber-Krum, S., Rohr, J., Kurutas, S., Karadon, D., Baykal, S. S., Okcuoglu, B. A., Esmer, Y., Canning, D., & Shah, I. (2021). Does cosmopolitan culture weaken ethnic and regional diversity: Contraceptive behaviors of women in Istanbul, Turkey. *The European Journal of Contraception & Reproductive Health Care: The Official Journal of the European Society of Contraception*, 1–7. Advance online publication. https://doi.org/10.1080/13625187.2021.1964466

   Agula, C., Henry, E. G., Asuming, P.O., Agyei-Asabere, C., Kushitor, M., Canning, D., Shah, I., & Bawah, A. A. (2021). Methods women use for induced abortion and sources of services: Insights from poor urban settlements of Accra, Ghana. *BMC Women's Health*, 21, 300. https://doi.org/10.1186/s12905-021-01444-9

   Henry, E. G., Agula, C., Agyei-Asabere, C., Asuming, P. O., Bawah, A. A., Canning, D., & Shah, I. (2021). Dynamics of emergency contraceptive use in Accra, Ghana. *Studies in Family Planning*, *52*(2), 105–123. https://doi.org/10.1111/sifp.12154

   Henry, E. G., Agula, C., Asuming, P. O., Kaur, N., Kruk, M., Shah, I., & Bawah, A. A. (2021). Conducting a household survey in poor urban settlements in Ghana: Challenges and strategic adaptations for fieldwork. *Journal of Global Health Science*, *3*(1). https://doi.org/10.35500/jghs.2021.3.e8

References

Ahmed, S., Li, Q., Liu, L., & Tsui, A. O. (2012). Maternal deaths averted by contraceptive use: An analysis of 172 countries. *The Lancet*, *380*(9837), 111–125. http://dx.doi.org/10.1016/S0140-6736(12)60478-4.

Bongaarts, J. (1984). Implications of future fertility trends for contraceptive practice. *Population and Development Review*, *10*(2), 341–352.

Bradley, S. E. K., Winfrey, W., & Croft, T. N. (2015). *Contraceptive use and perinatal mortality in the DHS: An assessment of the quality and consistency of calendars and histories*. DHS Methodological Reports. No. 17. ICF International.

Iacus, S. M., King, G., Porro, G., & Katz, J.N. (2012). Causal inference without balance checking: Coarsened exact matching. *Political Analysis, 20*(1), 1–24. doi:10.1093/pan/mpr013

Rupasinghe, N., Shah, I., Canning, D., & Sando, D. (forthcoming). *Community-based family planning interventions and contraceptive uptake: A systematic review.*

United Nations, Department of Economic and Social Affairs, Population Division (2020). *Estimates and projections of family planning indicators 2020.* United Nations.

DUYGU KARADON

5 Factors Influencing Reproductive Health Decision-Making

Abstract: This chapter aims at explaining how social, cultural, and especially religious factors influence willingness to seek knowledge of and the decision to actually use contraception with particular emphasis on modern methods and induced abortion. To delineate some of these determinants and better understand reproductive health decision-making processes, we conducted a qualitative study with 16 key informants in a diverse, low-income neighborhood of Istanbul, Turkey. The objective of the study was to better understand key actors' perceptions within the health care system and the community, and their willingness to share their own experiences and insights on reproductive health-related issues. Our findings show that multiple perspectives need to be considered for an adequate understanding of reproductive health decision-making processes, such as cultural norms, the role of male partners, social networks, sources of information, fatalism, and religious beliefs.

Keywords: Family planning, induced abortion, values, fertility norms, Turkish Demographic Health Survey, in-depth interviewing.

1 Introduction

It is not easy to address the question of what factors influence decision-making on reproductive health. Several factors have been suggested as predictors of family planning and abortion decision-making, and contributing factors vary for different cultures, values, and norms. At the same time, the accessibility and availability of contraception influence this decision-making process. The vast literature on the reproductive health decisions of individuals indicates that numerous aspects need to be taken into consideration as determinants of fertility preferences, contraceptive usage, and the decision to have an abortion, such as age, parity, level of education (Koç, 2000; Tadele et al., 2019; Seidu et al., 2020), urban or rural residence (Darteh et al., 2019), financial status (Cebeci Save et al., 2004; Rehnström Loi et al., 2018) and labor force participation (Finlay & Lee, 2018). In addition to these demographic characteristics, religious beliefs, social environment, power relations between couples (Orji et al., 2007) or within the family (Darteh et al., 2014), and even the sex of the living child/children (Koç, 2000) contribute to the decision-making process.

In the 1960s, Turkey adopted a national family planning policy to encourage traditional and modern contraceptive methods. Consequently, easy and free access to modern contraceptive methods and a range of reproductive health services became widespread. In 1983 (Law on Population Planning, 1983), Turkey further expanded this policy and proceeded to legalize induced abortions on request up to the first 10 weeks of pregnancy.

Although legally permitted, induced abortion services are not readily available due to certain legal restrictions and the unavailability of a full range of abortion services in public hospitals. Furthermore, public hospitals only provide abortion services if medically necessary. In addition, conservative social and cultural norms coupled with conservative Islamist government policies and rhetoric have complicated and hampered access to free and safe abortion services in the past 15 years.

Knowledge of contraception is universal. According to Turkish Demographic Health Survey (Hacettepe University Institute of Population Studies, 2019), 97 % of all women and 99 % of married women have heard about contraceptive methods. The most commonly used family planning methods are withdrawal (20 %), male condoms (19 %), IUDs (14 %), and female sterilization (10 %). Despite a high level of knowledge, approximately half of married women only use modern methods,[1] and a considerable proportion of women rely upon traditional methods[2] such as withdrawal.

The 2018 TDHS reported that 15 % of ever-married women have had one or more abortions during their lifetime. Although legal on request since the passing of the 1983 Act, abortion services are difficult for women to access in Turkey (MacFarlane et al., 2017; Telli et al., 2019). Legal restrictions such as the 10-week limitation, restriction of medical abortion pills, and the requirement of spousal/parental consent seem to be the primary barriers to accessing safe abortion services. Further, Turkey has no accurate or routine statistical data on unsafe abortions, and the ability to track any abortion information is limited. In addition, inducing an abortion on request is not permissible at public hospitals unless there is an endangerment to the mother's or fetus's life. Before the procedure is performed, the doctor must inform the health authorities about the women's identity, the procedure to be performed, and the justification for the abortion, which creates difficulty for women to access safe abortion services. Additional studies have shown that abortion is "legal but not necessarily available"[3] in Turkey. Few public hospitals provide abortion services on request, and many institutions do not offer abortion services. Additionally, 53 of Turkey's 81 provinces have no public hospital that offers elective abortion services (O'Neil, 2017).

TDHS indicates that the self-reported induced abortion rate has declined substantially over time. According to the results, the percentage of ever-married women (age 15–49 years) who had at least one induced abortion was 28 % in 1993 and 15 % in 2018. Another point to consider is that these estimations depend on direct questioning. Women's experiences of abortions during their lifetime are possibly underreported (Huber-Krum et al., 2020). The prevalence of abortion has decreased over the years, and the knowledge and use of modern contraception have increased. However, many women rely on traditional methods with high method failure rates, and many women report that one of the typical reasons for discontinuation is method failure (19 %).

Considering current health policies in Turkey, the purpose of the interviews was to better understand the perception of key actors related to the reproductive health decision-making process. To document country-specific variations in identifying potential contextual factors that may influence reproductive health issues, we interviewed 16 key informants. In-depth interviews were especially valuable due to increased privacy for participants who had been asked to discuss sensitive issues such as contraception and abortion. They provided insights into the barriers and facilitators in contraceptive decision-making, as well as perspectives on and experiences with unintended pregnancy and abortion.

2 Methodology

2.1 Study Design and Data Collection Procedures

In-depth interviews provided critical insights related to factors affecting contraceptive behavior, abortion prevalence, decision-making, care-seeking, and qualitative indication of opinions and lived experiences, which cannot be adequately captured by using quantitative methods. This qualitative in-depth interview study was conducted in Bağcılar, Istanbul, between April and May 2019. Bağcılar is a district of Istanbul, Turkey that has developed rapidly. Its population in 2019 was 745,125, according to the population count of the National Statistics Institute (TURKSTAT, 2019) based on addresses.

We used purposive sampling (Berg, 1995; Strauss & Corbin, 1998) and snowball sampling to recruit key informants. Examples of community stakeholders include religious leaders, neighborhood representatives, and local government members who had familiarity with reproductive health-related issues and potential influence in the community related to contraceptives and induced abortion behaviors. In total, we conducted 16 face-to-face interviews with family planning providers (8) and community stakeholders (8) in the study area. These interviews allowed us to gather further details on decision-making related to the reproductive health behaviors of women. Our sample of 16 participants was identified based on their potential role and potential impact on matters related to reproductive health and family planning issues.

All interviews were performed by the local field company that had experience in conducting qualitative studies. To generate a list of participants, the local field company and the research team worked together to identify potential participants. We selected family planning service providers from public and private hospitals that offered family planning and abortion services in the study area (Bağcılar, Istanbul) using a health facility survey conducted between August and October 2018. To formulate an interview schedule, the research team made several visits to Bağcılar.

Harvard University research team worked closely with the Turkish team to refine the interview guides and ensure a shared understanding of the objectives and research questions to be addressed through the interviews. All study tools (two semi-structured interview guides) were developed jointly in English and translated into Turkish for the interviews. The family planning service provider interview guide reviewed various points, including availability and quality of services, access to family planning and abortion services, perspectives on family planning and abortion for regulating fertility, and attitudes toward contraception and abortion. The community stakeholder interviewer guide addressed sociocultural norms and factors influencing access to family planning and abortion services, including community preferences and the behavior of women, which comprises gender norms and the decision-making of couples.

A trained female Turkish interviewer affiliated with the local field company conducted all interviews in Turkish. Before data collection, the interviewer participated in all training sessions, including sessions on ethical procedures, adherence to the ethical principles of informed choice, voluntary participation, privacy, and confidentiality. The interviewer conducted role-playing activities with the research team and was provided feedback. With the participants identified, the research team translated guidelines (one for family planning providers and one for community stakeholders) into Turkish and pilot tested two semi-structured interview guides (see selected key questions in Tab. 5.1).

Participants were free to refuse to answer any question in the interview guides or to withdraw entirely from the study at any time. Before each interview, the interviewer asked service providers and community stakeholders to provide oral[4] consent to take part in the study.

Interviews were conducted in quiet, private spaces to protect participant privacy. Interviews with family planning service providers took place in private rooms/offices within health facilities. Similarly, community stakeholder interviews were conducted in their house, which was convenient for participants. All interviews were audio-recorded with the permission of participants. Subsequently, audio recordings were transcribed verbatim in Turkish and translated into English. During this stage, all identifying information was removed from the transcripts before analysis. On average, interviews lasted approximately 60 minutes.

2.2 Analysis

We used Atlas-ti (Version 8.0) software for qualitative data management, coding, and analysis. We applied a multistage analytical (Strauss & Corbin, 1998) approach to develop preliminary key themes and a codebook for analysis. The grounded theory approach allowed flexibility for themes to emerge from the data rather than stringently applying pre-existing theories (Glaser & Strauss, 1967). Four researchers independently coded each transcript using the Atlas-ti software program. The team reviewed all transcripts and developed an initial list of codes. The codebook served as a reference that included definitions applicable to the reproductive health interviews.

Sixteen interviews were divided between four members of the research team, all codes were reviewed individually (more than 200 different codes), and open codes were applied to each transcript. Next, we developed a final codebook applicable to the key informant interviews, consisting of 51 subcodes within six main coding groups: background characteristics of participants, family planning, abortion, socially oriented perspectives, quality of services, and reproductive health programs. Finally, the research team double-coded all interviews to improve the quality of the analysis.

Tab. 5.1: Selected key questions from semi-structured key informant interview guides

Family Planning Provider	
Availability and quality of reproductive health services	➢ Can you tell me about the reproductive health services available at this facility? ➢ What do you think most influences women's desire to use modern family planning methods? ➢ Can you tell me about the demand for family planning and abortion services in this area?
Experiences providing reproductive health services at this facility	➢ Generally, how do you feel about providing family planning services? ➢ Can you think of any situations in the past in which you were not comfortable providing reproductive health services?
Community Stakeholders	
Availability and quality of reproductive health services	➢ Can you tell me about the demand for family planning and abortion that you observe in your community? ➢ Where (or to whom) do most people go to obtain family planning information? ➢ What does the local community think about family planning in general? ➢ What does the local community think about abortion in general?

3 Results

3.1 Selected Background Characteristics of Participants

The selected background characteristics of the participants are summarized in Tab. 5.2. Family planning providers in our sample include six physicians/gynecologists and two midwives. Overall, service providers had been providing family planning services for between one and 22 years. Concerning the community stakeholders, two were affiliated with Adalet ve Kalkinma Partisi (the conservative and ruling party since 2002), two were local parent-teacher association members/representatives, one was a local prayer group leader, and one was the assistant of a neighborhood representative. In addition, one community stakeholder was a pharmacist, and another was a pharmacist's assistant. The pharmacist and the pharmacist's assistant were considered community stakeholders, as they frequently provide informal consultation, guidance, and advice to women about fertility planning and reproductive health.

Tab. 5.2: Selected background characteristics of participants

Participant Number	Participant Type	Gender	Community role/ Current position	Years in current position	Years providing family planning services
1	Community stakeholder	Female	Ak Parti member and Parent-teacher association member	–	–
2	Community stakeholder	Female	Prayer group leader	–	–
3	Community stakeholder	Female	Pharmacist	36 years	–
4	Community stakeholder	Female	Pharmacy assistant	20 years	–
5	Community stakeholder	Female	Neighborhood representative's assistant	–	–
6	Family planning provider	Female	Physician	8.5 years	8.5 years
7	Family planning provider	Female	Midwife	14 years	14 years
8	Community stakeholder	Female	Parent- teacher association member	–	–
9	Family planning provider	Male	Gynecologist	20 years	20 years
10	Family planning provider	Female	Gynecologist	14 years	22 years
11	Community stakeholder	Female	Ak Parti neighborhood representative	–	–
12	Community stakeholder	Female	Parent- teacher association member	–	–
13	Family planning provider	Female	Gynecologist	1 year	1 year
14	Family planning provider	Female	Midwife	10 years	10 years
15	Family planning provider	Female	Gynecologist	4 months	7 years
16	Family planning provider	Female	Gynecologist	17 years	17 years

3.2 Themes in Qualitative Data

Theme development followed an inductive approach, using themes that emerged from the data. In that study, four key themes arose from the transcripts corresponding to the decision-making process (related to either family planning or abortion). Table 5.3 outlines four primary themes, including participation in decision-making, the influence of male partners, sources of information, and the impact of religious beliefs, along with definitions and examples.

Tab. 5.3: Definition and examples of key themes

Themes	Definition	Verbatim quotation
Participation in decision-making	Mentions of decision-making involvement (e.g., freedom to choose any traditional or modern method to use, abortion demand and access).	*Because they [women] don't want to get pregnant. It is always the women who endure the hardships of pregnancy, so they make the decisions.* (Interviewee 11, Community stakeholder)
The influence of male partners	Demand for family planning/ abortion and discussions related to family size, formation, childbearing spacing.	*There are some women who don't use birth control because they are afraid of their husbands.* (Interviewee 2, Community stakeholder)
Source of information	Any discussion about family planning and induced abortion with friends, family members, neighbors (e.g., trade-off thinking, advice, rumors).	*The women here generally don't go to the health center, they talk among themselves; "How do you manage birth control?" or "I use this, if it is good I will use that." If I recommend, if it works for her, it will work for me too.* (Interviewee 2, Community stakeholder)
The impact of religious beliefs	Impact of religious beliefs on contraception and abortion (e.g., barriers to using or accessing any family planning/ abortion services).	*They [people in the community] are against it [family planning] because of religious reasons.* (Interviewee 9, Family planning provider)

3.3 Participation in Decision-making

In general, most participants agreed that there was a substantial demand for modern contraceptive services among women. Many participants discussed the increasing awareness of women about modern contraceptive methods, particularly among young women who wanted to delay or space childbearing and among women who wished to limit births. The growing demand for modern contraception seemed to reflect a growing desire to delay birth during adolescence and young adulthood and limit birth after women had achieved their ideal family size. The providers' narratives implied that they were supportive of these growing trends and actively encouraged young women to meet their reproductive goals, whether that be through the use of modern contraception or healthy preconception and birth planning.

Respondents differed with regard to what methods they believed to be most popular among women. Although they agreed that a number of modern contraceptive methods were available and used by women in Bağcılar, many also agreed that traditional family planning methods, such as withdrawal and periodic abstinence, were preferred due to the lack of side effects and the convenience of use.

Across the interviews, almost all participants shared the view that it is women who decide whether to prevent pregnancy or not. Hence, family planning decisions are considered a woman's domain by service providers and community stakeholders.

> *... women have to think about [birth control] as they are the ones who take care of the children. So the women make the decisions. (Interviewee 8, Community stakeholder)*
> *Because they [women] don't want to get pregnant. It is always the women who endure the hardships of pregnancy, so they make the decisions. (Interviewee 11, Community stakeholder)*

While family planning decisions are usually perceived as a woman's domain, in some cases these decisions are regarded as family decisions. Few participants reported that family planning decisions (either to use or not use a method) were made by family members, including in-laws. A family planning service provider said:

> *I had a few clients whose mothers-in-law wanted their daughters-in-law to have more children. And this affects the spouses or the husbands, and they think about having another child. As they live together, the mother-in-law or even the father-in-law influences [their decisions to have another child]. (Interviewee 6, Family planning provider)*

Regarding abortion, all respondents agreed that there is a very low prevalence of induced abortion among women in their communities. Many community stakeholders reported that they had "*never heard of it happening.*" Although family planning providers seemed to be much more aware of abortion incidence, they also agreed that few women obtain abortions through formal healthcare settings. Additionally, service providers who are unwilling to perform abortions frequently referred to anti-abortion discourse such as "*every life is valued*" and "*abortion is murder*" (Interviewee 9, Family planning provider). Another community stakeholder reported the following:

I have never heard of abortion here for the last 10 years… never. There used to be abortion services, but I have never heard of it. (Interviewee 11, Community stakeholder)

The availability of abortion services to women was one of the most discussed topics in the study. Many service providers stated their opposition to elective abortion. They prefer not to perform induced abortions on request because of their personal, religious, or cultural beliefs, even though abortion is allowed at the health facility where they work. Biased thoughts and behaviors about abortion from family planning service providers described the following comments:

I do not end healthy pregnancies; this is my principle. I have never done it. We do it if it is a medical necessity. We respect every living thing. But if the baby has some serious defect like an undeveloped head, or if there is an incomplete miscarriage, we will help them end the pregnancy, of course. But if it's perfectly healthy, I will not do it. I think I would feel uneasy about it. It is a life, after all, and I do not want to be the one who takes it. (Interviewee 13, family planning provider)

If the baby's heartbeat has stopped or the mother has had an incomplete miscarriage, [an abortion] can be performed… But it has to be a medical necessity. Elective abortion is not available, as the hospital management does not want it. (Interviewee 15, family planning provider)

3.4 Influence of Male Partners

The majority of respondents reported that there was a higher demand for modern contraceptive services by women than men. Many respondents noted that men were not in favor of modern contraceptive methods and had very limited involvement with family planning matters. However, it did not seem as though men actively objected to using modern contraception. It was clear from participants' narratives (both service providers and community stakeholders) that family planning remains a woman's domain, which generally means that women determine whether or not to end pregnancies. Family planning providers reported that it is rare for male partners to escort women to appointments, although men would be welcomed to join if the woman wanted. Community stakeholders agreed that women also do not trust men to be included in decisions on family planning. The following comment described the situation: "*Men are not trusted to be involved with family planning by women. Men are fine with* [women's decisions] …*I think this responsibility is given to the women in Turkey*" (Interviewee 15, Family planning provider). Additionally, most respondents agreed that men have strong opposition to induced abortion. A gynecologist who has provided family planning services for 20 years said, "*Men do not want an abortion. And they do not want to use birth control. They want children even if it is the fifteenth child*" (Interviewee 9, family planning provider).

The lack of male involvement in family planning decision-making also seemed to derive from pro-natalist opinions. Participants noted that men are more likely to desire many children and thus may not see value in contraceptive use. Further, the burden of childrearing responsibilities seemed to fall on women across all interviews. Thus, men were reported to simply "*not care*" about contraceptive use:

> *When [women] bear a child, most husbands do not help with childcare. It is as if the child belongs only to the mother; supposedly, he is the father. When the child is sick, the mother takes care of him/her; and when the mother is sick, the father cannot take care of the child… Men generally say that they are unable to take care of children. So, women want birth control methods to avoid consecutive births.* (Interviewee 14, Family planning provider)
>
> *Because they [men] don't care about having a lot of children as they don't look after them.* (Interviewee 5, Community stakeholder)

The use of contraceptive methods without husbands' knowledge was one of the most frequently discussed topics across all transcripts. Related to readily concealed strategies that cannot easily be noticed by male partners, such as pills and IUDs, most participants shared these views:

> *There are some women who do not use birth control because they are afraid of their husbands…They use the pills, I mean they use the pills secretly without letting their husbands know. Most of them don't prefer injections, so they use the pills. They get the pills from the health centers, and they use them by not telling their husbands. (Interviewee 5, Community stakeholder)*
>
> *…especially the husbands want more children, so the women sometimes get these [family planning methods] without telling their husbands.* (Interviewee 3, Community stakeholder)

3.5 Sources of Information

All respondents stated that modern contraceptive methods are easily accessible and available at hospitals and pharmacies. Further, most participants noted that methods are easily accessible from health facilities as well as that women trust healthcare providers and the information they receive from them. Several respondents noted that rumors about contraception, while present, were not to be believed.

Women did seem to obtain information about contraception from their friends but often verified this information with a healthcare professional before making any decisions about whether to use contraception. A midwife who had been in her position for 10 years reported the following:

I think the people who get family planning services need to be educated. In terms of the cultural structure, most of the people, especially in this neighborhood, are uneducated. They come here (i.e., to the health facility) to get help with secondhand information, with other people's recommendation… They say that their neighbors use the IUD and are very satisfied, so they want to use it, too. They need to be educated. (Interviewee 14, Family planning provider)

Women rely more on information from secondary sources and advice they have received. Meanwhile, a few respondents discussed the impact of secondhand information as a prevalent choice.

First, they [women] talk among themselves. For example, she asks me how I manage birth control, how I prevent pregnancy. I say that I use the pill or injections or that my husband uses a method. She says that if it is good, she will do it too. Then, she goes to the health center to ask the nurses… It is the culture of the women here, nothing else. It is better for them to hear it instead of searching and learning, I think. As women we are like this, we don't want to improve ourselves. We can if we try but still "If Ayşe is using that, Fatma can use that too." But actually it is wrong. We have doctors, nurses, health centers, midwives, but still we don't go. It is the last resort. (Interviewee 1, Community stakeholder)

Another participant also described how women could have miscarriages outside of formal healthcare centers based on received advice:

The neighbor is the midwife, a midwife in the village. She doesn't have a certificate or anything, but she knows how to deliver babies. So they go and ask her or do what they can to have a miscarriage … Actually there was one. She didn't want to have an abortion at the hospital, so she was trying at home by lifting heavy things or using some pills to have bleeding. (Interviewee 1, Community stakeholder)

3.6 Impact of Religious Beliefs

Few barriers to contraception were reported by participants, and their narratives suggested relatively few reasons for the nonuse of contraception. However, a frequent argument that also overlapped with barriers to abortion was the importance of religious beliefs on reproductive health decisions. Several respondents stated that women considered modern contraception, in general, or specific methods to be a sin. A family planning service provider reported that:

Actually, there is a prejudice against most of the birth control methods in our society … It is considered as a sin. They don't want birth control. The woman doesn't want the IUD. They use the withdrawal method, but it is not a birth control method. They see it as a method, but we have a lot of patients coming here for an unplanned pregnancy. If they were informed beforehand, it would affect the consequences, of course. (Interviewee 13, Family planning provider)

Additionally, a parent-teacher association member said the following:

> *Some spouses consider [birth control] as a sin. We hear it from our friends... For example, the woman wants to use birth control, but the husband thinks it is a sin and they do not use anything.* (Interviewee 8, Community stakeholder)

Religious norms also seemed to deter women from having abortions. Further, there may be a low prevalence of abortion due to the social value of pregnancy and social norms of pregnancy fatalism. Often discussed concurrently with religious opposition to abortion, expressed by the majority of respondents themselves or of women in their communities, is the belief that pregnancy is predetermined and therefore inevitable. Further, pregnancy fatalism seemed to be more prevalent among younger women who may be more likely to fear physical, social, or religious consequences of using contraception or abortion. The quotes below highlight these fatalistic beliefs:

> *Getting pregnant and then having an abortion is very bad because of physical, mental and religious reasons. So if God has given it, we must consent.* (Interviewee 8, Community stakeholder)
> *The people believe that if God gives the baby, God will help them ... you cannot take away what God gives.* (Interviewee 3, Community stakeholder)

4 Discussion

This qualitative data was not without limitations. Community stakeholders at the study site were purposively selected following their familiarity with women's sexual and reproductive health matters along with family planning and abortion. Furthermore, the gender diversity of the participants was another limitation since there was only one male respondent. Because participants were purposively selected to be part of the study, it is impossible to generalize the study's results to the entire population.

The study's focus was on the reproductive health decision-making process, including family planning and abortion; in-depth interviews enabled us to understand the evolution of the opinions of members of the community and providers. Findings from qualitative data illustrate key factors and determinants that influence those decisions. There is general contraceptive knowledge in Turkey. According to the last TDHS (2018), 99 % of currently married women (women aged 15–49) know of at least one contraceptive method, either modern or traditional. The research findings are in accordance with existing family planning literature considering a high level of knowledge of contraceptive methods in the community. Key informants reported that, compared to modern methods, women tend to prefer traditional methods. According to their perception of women in the study area, the most influential factors in choosing a contraceptive method are the ease of use and lack of side effects. Modern contraceptive methods are commonly considered to have undesired side effects; therefore, traditional methods are preferred when deciding which method to use. In addition, family planning decision-making was perceived as a woman's domain since they shouldered the primary responsibility for childcare; however, other family members, such as in-laws, may also engage in the decision-making process.

Drawing from participants' narratives, there is a low prevalence of abortion. This may be related to underreporting abortion behaviors related to inaccessibility, providers' reluctance, biased thoughts and behaviors about abortion, and ignorance of abortion laws (Huber-Krum et al., 2020), suggesting that the phenomenon of very low prevalence may be widespread. Furthermore, according to TDHS (2018), 62 % of women decided to have an induced abortion with service providers' advice, which refers to the medical necessity of obtaining safe abortion services. Additional studies are essential to explain how women obtain an abortion in Istanbul.

The role of male partners in reproductive health decision-making has been demonstrated in several prior studies. Some believe it is a shared responsibility that refers to participating in decision-making jointly (e.g., Mistik et al., 2003; Şahin, 2008; Zeyneloğlu et al., 2013). Conversely, many findings suggest that neither men nor women are generally opposed to family planning methods (either modern and traditional methods), yet women are perceived as the ones who determine reproductive health-related issues (Angin & Shorter, 1998; Cebeci Save et al., 2004). In this study, many respondents believed that men were not currently involved in contraceptive decision-making and modern contraceptive use was primarily a woman's domain. Although some participants indicated that men might be resistant to contraceptive usage, the majority stated that men were merely indifferent and unconcerned about birth control. In short, there is a lack of male involvement in family planning issues, and male partners desire more children than women. Additionally, men are strongly opposed to abortion. In these circumstances, they have a pro-natalist opinion since it is generally women who suffer the emotional and physical impacts of having many children.

Globally, many women favor the discreet use of contraception without their partner's knowledge. Poor information, mistrust, poor quality of communication, and conflict between spouses about family planning may all motivate women to use contraceptives covertly (Biddlecom & Fapohunda, 1998; Baiden et al., 2016). Oral contraceptives, emergency contraception, injectables, and IUDs are the preferred modern methods that can be easily concealed (Koenig et al.,1984). Previous studies have investigated some aspects of covert contraceptive use, and findings from the present study also highlight the prevalence of covert contraceptive use among women.

Both family planning service providers and community stakeholders agreed that women trust service providers. However, the source of the information cannot be discounted in reproductive health decision-making. Our participants mostly agreed that women tend to believe secondhand recommendations/information based on the previous experiences of their friends, relatives, or neighbors. This emphasizes the importance of social networks for women both as a source of information and as a determinant of behavior. Other studies suggest that the source of information is essential in reproductive health decision-making, specifically about the method of choice, side effects, convenience in use, safety, and effectiveness. Many women assume that secondhand knowledge is more accurate than any other source of information (Yee & Simon, 2010).

Religious beliefs were one of the most discussed topics, either related to contraceptive usage or abortion. Further, respondents and their community members displayed fatalistic beliefs about pregnancy and birth. Pregnancy fatalism has been documented in societies across the globe and may result in the failure to use contraception or the failure to use contraception correctly (e.g., Çavlin et al., 2012; Jones et al., 2016; Jones, 2018). However, qualitative studies of pregnancy fatalism also reveal that it may not reduce or remove the motivation to use contraception, only that fatalistic beliefs can act as a coping mechanism for unplanned pregnancies or unrealized fertility (Jones, 2018). High levels of modern contraceptive use can coexist with the presence of fatalism and negative beliefs about contraception, as documented elsewhere (Jones, 2018; Machiyama et al., 2018). However, our qualitative data reveal that pregnancy fatalism may deter women from preventing unwanted births through abortion services, specifically. As Jones et al. (2016) note, many women do not actually have total control of pregnancy prevention. Thus, pregnancy fatalism should be viewed as a pragmatic response to cope with an unplanned pregnancy. Further, women can hold fatalistic views about pregnancy but also use contraception, and nonuse of contraception could be an indication of ambivalence about pregnancy (Jones, 2018).

5 Conclusion

In-depth interviews with service providers and community stakeholders were critical to address broader perspectives about the decision-making process related to women's family planning and abortion attitudes in the community. The qualitative study provided new insights into aspects of fertility regulation using contraception and abortion. Reproductive health decision-making is multilayered. Hence, it is not possible to identify a single explanation to entirely understand this process. The findings indicate that women are the decision-makers in reproductive health-related issues, while men keep a distance from family planning matters and are typically not involved in contraceptive decision-making. On the other hand, women trust healthcare service providers and the information that they receive from them but might rely more on the experiences of other people.

Further, family planning service providers note that only a limited number of women avail themselves of safe abortion services. Cultural and social norms as well as provider biases seem to be the primary barriers to accessing safe abortion services. We note that abortion is perceived as unjustifiable by large segments of society, and people have deep-running fatalistic attitudes toward family planning and abortion methods. Cultural, social and religious norms and values are determinants of reproductive matters, including the decision-making process, accessibility, and availability. From this perspective, any study or analysis will be incomplete without considering this approach.

Notes

1. Female sterilization, male sterilization, intrauterine devices (IUDs), injectables, implants, female condoms, male condoms, pills, diaphragm/foam/jelly, vaginal ring, emergency contraception (EC), standard days method, and Lactational amenorrhea (LAM) (Festin et al., 2016)
2. Withdrawal, rhythm and other traditional methods (Festin et al., 2016)
3. *Legal but Not Necessarily Available: Abortion Services at State Hospitals in Turkey* (O'Neil et al., 2016) is the title of the research project at the Gender and Women's Studies Research Center at Kadir Has University.
4. Collecting written consent was inappropriate due to security concerns.

References

Angin, Z., & Shorter, F. C. (1998). Negotiating reproduction and gender during the fertility decline in Turkey. *Social Science & Medicine*, *47*(5), 555–564.

Baiden, F., Mensah, G. P., Akoto, N. O., Delvaux, T., & Appiah, P. C. (2016). Covert contraceptive use among women attending a reproductive health clinic in a municipality in Ghana. *BMC Women's Health*, *16*(31). https://doi.org/10.1186/s12905-016-0310-x

Berg, B. L. (1995). *Qualitative research methods for the social sciences* (2nd ed.). Allyn and Bacon.

Biddlecom, A. E., & Fapohunda, B. M. (1998). Covert contraceptive use: Prevalence, motivations, and consequences. *Studies in Family Planning, 29*(4), 360.

Cebeci Save, D., Erbaydar, T., Kalaca, S., Harmancı, H., Çalı, S., & Karavuş, M. (2004). Resistance against contraception or medical contraceptive methods: A qualitative study on women and men in Istanbul. *The European Journal of Contraception & Reproductive Health Care, 9*(2), 94–101.

Çavlin, A., Tezcan, S., & Ergöçmen, B. (2012). Kadınların bakış açısından kürtaj. *Turkish Journal of Population Studies, 34*, 51–67.

Darteh, E. K. M., Doku, D. T., & Esia-Donkoh, K. (2014). Reproductive health decision making among Ghanaian women. *Reproductive Health, 11*(23), 1–8.

Darteh, E. K. M., Dickson, K. S., & Doku, D. T. (2019). Women's reproductive health decision-making: A multi-country analysis of demographic and health surveys in sub-Saharan Africa. *PLOS ONE, 14*(1).

Festin, M. P. R., Kiarie, J., Solo, J., Spieler, J., Malarcher, S., Van Look, P. F. A., & Temmerman, M. (2016). Moving towards the goals of FP2020 - Classifying contraceptives. *Contraception, 94*(4), 289–294.

Finlay, J. E., & Lee, M. A. (2018). Identifying causal effects of reproductive health improvements on women's economic empowerment through the population poverty research initiative. *The Milbank Quarterly, 96*(2), 300–322.

Glaser, B., & Strauss, A. (1967). *The discovery of Grounded Theory*. Chicago: Aldine.

Hacettepe University Institute of Population Studies. (2019). *Turkey Demographic and Health Survey 2018*. https://dhsprogram.com/pubs/pdf/FR372/FR372.pdf.

Huber-Krum, S., Karadon, D., Kurutaş, S., Rohr, J., Baykal, S. S., Okçuoglu, B. A., Esmer, Y., Canning, D., & Shah, I. (2020). Estimating abortion prevalence and understanding perspectives of community leaders and providers: Results from a mixed-method study in Istanbul, Turkey. *Women's Health, 16*, 1–13.

Jones, R. K. (2018). Is pregnancy fatalism normal? An attitudinal assessment among women trying to get pregnant and those not using contraception. *Contraception, 98*(4), 255- 259.

Jones, R. K., Frohwirth, L. F., & Blades, N. M. (2016). "If I know I am on the pill and I get pregnant, it's an act of God": Women's views on fatalism, agency and pregnancy. *Contraception, 93*(6), 551–555.

Koç, I. (2000). Determinants of contraceptive use and method choice in Turkey. *Journal of Biosocial Science, 32*(3), 329–342.

Koenig, M. A., Simmons, G. B., & Misra, B. D. (1984). Husband – Wife inconsistencies in contraceptive use responses. *Population Studies*, *38*(2), 281–298.

Law on Population Planning No. 2827 (1983), Retrieved from http://www.mevzuat.gov.tr/MevzuatMetin/1.5.2827.pdf

MacFarlane, K. A., O'Neil, M. L., Tekdemir, D., & Foster, A.M. (2017). It was as if society didn't want a woman to get an abortion: a qualitative study in Istanbul, Turkey. *Contraception*, *95*(2), 154–160.

Machiyama, K., Huda, F. A., Ahmmed, F., Odwe, G., Obare, F., Mumah, J. N., Wamukoya, M., Casterline, J. B., & Cleland, J. (2018). Women's attitudes and beliefs towards specific contraceptive methods in Bangladesh and Kenya. *Reproductive Health*, *15*(1), 75.

Mistik, S., Naçar, M., Mazicioğlu, M., & Çetinkaya, F. (2003). Married men's opinions and involvement regarding family planning in rural areas. *Contraception*, *67*, 133–137.

National Statistics Institute (TURKSTAT). (2019). Retrieved February 3, 2020 from https://biruni.tuik.gov.tr/medas/?kn=95&locale=tr

O'Neil, M. L., Aldanmaz, B., Quiles, R. M. Q., & Kılınç, F. R. (2016). Legal but not necessarily available: Abortion services at state hospitals in Turkey. https://gender.khas.edu.tr/sites/gender.khas.edu.tr/files/inline-files/Abortion%20English.pdf.

O'Neil, M. L. (2017). Abortion services at hospitals in Istanbul. *The European Journal of Contraception & Reproductive Health Care*, *22*(2), 88–93.

Orji, E. O., Ojofeitimi, E. O., & Olanrewaju, B. A. (2007). The role of men in family planning decision-making in rural and urban Nigeria, *The European Journal of Contraception & Reproductive Health Care*, *12*(1), 70–75.

Rehnström Loi, U., Lindgren, M., Faxelid, E., Oguttu, M., & Klingberg-Allvin, M. (2018). Decision-making preceding induced abortion: A qualitative study of women's experiences in Kisumu, Kenya. *Reproductive Health*, *15*(166). https://doi.org/10.1186/s12978-018-0612-6

Seidu, A.-A., Ahinkorah, B. O., Ameyaw, E. K., Hubert, A., Agbemavi, W., Armah-Ansah, E.K., Budu, E., Sambah, F., & Tackie, V. (2020). What has women's reproductive health decision-making capacity and other factors got to do with pregnancy termination in sub-Saharan Africa? Evidence from 27 cross-sectional surveys. *PLOS ONE*, *15*(7), 1–17.

Strauss, A., & Corbin, J. (1998). *Basics of qualitative research: Techniques and procedures for developing grounded theory*. SAGE Publications.

Şahin, N. H. (2008). Male university students' views, attitudes and behaviors towards family planning and emergency contraception in Turkey. *The Journal of Obstetrics and Gynaecology Research*, *34*(3), 392–398.

Tadele, A., Tesfay, A., & Kebede, A. (2019). Factors influencing decision-making power regarding reproductive health and rights among married women in Mettu rural district, south-west, Ethiopia. *Reproductive Heath*, *16*(155), 1–9.

Telli, P., Cesuroğlu, T., & Tanık, F. A. (2019). How do pronatalist policies impact women's access to safe abortion services in Turkey? *International Journal of Health Services*, *49*(4), 799–816.

Yee, L. M., & Simon, M. (2010). The role of the social network in contraceptive decision- making among young, African American and Latina women. *Journal of Adolescent Health*, *47*(4), 374–380.

Zeyneloğlu, S., Kısa, S., & Delibaş, L. (2013). Determinants of family planning use among Turkish married men who live in South East Turkey. *American Journal of Men's Health*, *7*(3), 255–264.

SARAH HUBER-KRUM

6 Ethnic and Regional Diversity in Family Planning Behaviors

Abstract: The primary aim of the chapter is to examine the relationship between self-reported ethnic identity and contraceptive method use in urban Istanbul, Turkey. We analyzed cross-sectional data from a random sample of 3,038 married women of reproductive age, collected as part of an impact evaluation of a family planning intervention in two urban districts of Istanbul. We used a series of logistic regression models to assess key relationships, accounting for survey design. Kurdish women were less likely than Turkish women to use traditional methods over no method. However, there were no significant differences between ethnicities and modern method use. Among Turkish women, those born in regions further away from the Western region had a greater risk of using traditional methods. Among only Kurdish women, living in their neighborhood for less time was associated with reduced risk of using traditional or modern methods, compared to no method. While Kurdish women were less likely to use traditional methods than Turkish women, this difference may be due to other factors, namely time living in one's neighborhood. Regional traditions of traditional method use may be a barrier to modern contraceptive use in Turkey.

Keywords: Modern contraceptives, traditional contraceptive methods, ethnicity and contraceptive use, unintended pregnancy.

1 Introduction

Unintended pregnancy is a common phenomenon across low- and middle-income countries (LMICs): the average annual unintended pregnancy rate was approximately 80 pregnancies per 1,000 women aged 15–49 years in 2015–2019 (Bearak et al., 2020, pp. 1990–2019). The greatest contributor to unintended pregnancy is nonuse of modern contraception. Approximately 56 % of women who experienced an unintended pregnancy between 2005 and 2014 did not use any family planning in the past 5 years; almost 10 % of women who experienced an unintended pregnancy last used a traditional method (Bellizzi et al., 2020), such as withdrawal or rhythm method.

Disparities in modern contraceptive use may be partially attributed to differences in race and ethnicity. Most evident are those observed in high-income countries. For example, in the U.S., racial and ethnic minority women are more likely to experience unintended pregnancy and are less likely to use contraception (Dehlendorf et al., 2014; Grady et al., 2015). The type of contraceptive method used may also vary by race and ethnicity (Dehlendorf et al., 2011; Grady et al., 2015). Hypothesized mechanisms for differences in contraceptive use by race and ethnicity include differential socioeconomic status, fertility norms, and under-utilization of healthcare; however, some studies provide evidence that these factors make no difference (Dehlendorf et al., 2014). Other potential reasons for these disparities in the U.S. include system-level factors, such as differential access to health care services (Armstrong et al., 2007; Kennedy et al., 2007) and differences in the quality of family planning care (Becker & Tsui, 2008). Individual-level factors, such as differences in patient knowledge, preferences, cultural norms, concerns about modern contraception, and social mobility, may also contribute to these observed variations (Dehlendorf et al., 2011; Guendelman et al., 2000; Sangi-Haghpeykar et al., 2006).

Despite that health disparities often exist between ethnic majority and minority populations in LMICs, variations in the use of reproductive health services have not been as consistently investigated across a range of settings (Brockerhoff & Hewett, 2000). However, studies suggest that ethnic minority women are consistently less likely to use family planning compared to their ethnic majority counterparts. For example, self-identified indigenous women who live in the northeastern Ch'orti area of Guatemala are less likely than women who identified themselves as Ladino or "mixed" to use any family planning method (De Broe et al., 2005). Indigenous women in Bolivia are also less likely than nonindigenous women to use any family planning method (McNamee, 2009). Ethnic minority women in Nepal (e.g., Muslim, Dalit and Madhesi) are less likely to use modern contraception than ethnic majority women (i.e., Brahmin/Chhetri) (Mishra, 2010). Potential reasons for these variations among ethnic groups in LMICs may be similar to those seen in the U.S., such as system-level barriers to health care (De Broe et al., 2005) and individual-level cultural and norms-related barriers (McNamee, 2009; Mishra, 2010). However, the underlying mechanisms that contribute to these disparities are poorly understood.

In this study, we examined the relationship between self-reported ethnicity and use of family planning methods in Turkey, a multi-ethnic and multi-lingual country that straddles Southeastern Europe and West Asia. Kurds are the largest ethnic minority in Turkey, comprising about 19 % of the population (Central Intelligence Agency, 2020). Turks are the predominante ethnic majority, comprising about 70–75 % of the population (Central Intelligence Agency, 2020). Kurdish people live throughout Turkey. However, they are primarily concentrated in the Eastern and Southeastern regions that is considered a part of Turkish Kurdistan. Internal migration is common, but most often internal migrants move from the Eastern and Southeastern regions, which border Armenia, Iran, Iraq, Syria, to the Western region in which Istanbul is located (Saatçi & Akpınar, 2007). The Eastern region was also home to a large population of Armenians until the Armenian Genocide of 1915 and was called Western Armenia until the early 1920s. In the Southeast region, some provinces (e.g., Mardin) have a history of internal conflict between major ethnic and religious groups, such as that between Kurds and Arabs. As a whole, the Eastern regions have historically experienced higher fertility rates compared to the rest of Turkey (Yüceşahin & Özgür, 2008) and less likely to use modern contraception (Erman & Behrman, 2019), suggesting that ethnicity and cultural factors play a role in family planning behaviors.

The Turkish-Kurdish conflict is relatively long-standing, dating back to the formation of the Republic of Turkey. The government aspired to create a homogenous nation-state that emphasized Turkish language and identity (Arslan, 2015), and thus, some ethnic minorities groups – particularly Kurdish populations – resisted these efforts. The European Court of Human Rights has condemned Turkey for human rights abuses against Kurdish peoples, which include forced displacement (European Court of Human Rights, 2015; Human Rights Watch, 2006). Consequently, the Turkish government rarely acknowledges the Kurdish minority, resulting in surveys not collecting data about self-reported ethnicity. As an alternative to data on ethnicity, region of birth or cohabitation are used as proxies to explain differences in socioeconomic indicators or health disparities (Saatçi & Akpınar, 2007). Additionally, Kurdish identity is complex. Some individuals might identify as Kurdish without reading, writing, or verbal proficiency in the Kurdish language, while others might identify as Turkish and can speak Kurdish (Arslan, 2015). Since most government services are provided in the Turkish language, some individuals who only speak Kurdish or speak only little Turkish may have difficulty accessing services (Sulaivany, 2019).

The relationship between ethnic identity, region, and internal migration is complex in Turkey. In this paper, we also examined the association between contraceptive use and region of birth and time living in one's neighborhood. Region of birth has been used in past studies in Turkey as a proxy for ethnic differences; given the differential history of the seven regions of Turkey, regional differences in healthcare utilization are possible that persist even after migration to an urban hub. Additionally, the history of forced displacement among ethnic minority groups, especially among Kurdish populations, and the common trend of internal migration from the Eastern and Southeastern regions to Istanbul, time living in one's neighborhood may be indicative of conformity to other cultures' norms in an urban setting (i.e., assimilation or acculturation). Residing in

Istanbul may have an influence on converging contraceptive behaviors of diverse ethnic groups. In other words, as diverse groups live closer to one another, their behaviors may become more similar over time.

Our study addresses two existing research gaps. First, our study provides evidence about the relationship between self-report ethnicity and contraceptive use in Turkey, a topic that is understudied. The Turkey Demographic and Health Survey (TDHS), the largest, nationally representative survey of sexual and reproductive health in Turkey, does not ask about self-reported ethnic identity; however, TDHS does ask about languages spoken, such as Turkish, Kurdish, and Arabic, and researchers have used language as a proxy for ethnicity. Second, we consider how region of birth and time living in one's neighborhood is also associated with contraceptive use, providing a more complete picture of reproductive health disparities in urban Istanbul.

2 Methods

2.1 Setting and Study Design

Between March and June 2018, we conducted a cross-sectional household survey with married women of aged 15–44 years living in the communities of Bağcılar and Küçükçekmece, Istanbul. The survey study was part of an impact evaluation of the Willow's International Reproductive Health Program in Turkey. This research was approved by the ethical review board of Bahçeşehir University, and by the Institutional Review Board at Harvard University.

Bağcılar and Küçükçekmece (both located west of Istanbul city center) are comprised of diverse, low-income populations. The neighborhoods are large, with over 700,000 residents, and attract many migrants from Eastern and Southeastern Anatolia. As compared to married women aged 15–49 who lived in the Istanbul region, smaller proportions of women in our study sample used modern contraceptive methods (37 % in our study sample compared to 51 % in the 2018 TDHS (Hacettepe University Institute of Population Studies, 2019)), but slightly larger proportions reported use of any family planning method (72 % in our study sample compared to 69 % reported in the 2018 TDHS (Hacettepe University Institute of Population Studies, 2019)). In terms of background characteristics, married women in our sample were less educated and older compared to all women nationally (Hacettepe University Institute of Population Studies, 2019).

A minimum sample size of 4,000 women (2,000 in Bağcılar and 2,000 in Küçükçekmece) was predetermined based on a power calculation in our main outcome, the modern contraceptive prevalence rate, to give a 0.9 probability of being able to detect a five percentage point difference between the study sites. Using the National Statistics Institute (TURKSTAT) address list, we randomly sampled streets in each site. In total, 166 streets out of 296 streets were sampled in Bağcılar, and 87 streets out of 101 streets were sampled in Küçükçekmece. For streets with more than 100 households in Bağcılar or more than 200 households in Küçükçekmece, households were randomly sampled. Two hundred households, rather than 100, were selected in Küçükçekmece due to the slightly larger size of the community. In Bağcılar, there were 36 sampled street with more than 100 households; we randomly selected 100 households. In Küçükçekmece, there were 29 sampled streets with more than 200 households; we randomly selected 200 households. In total, 9,664 households in Bağcılar and 8,934 households in Küçükçekmece were randomly sampled. Some households refused the interview or were not available, resulting in 5,276 households reached in Bağcılar and 4,787 households reached in Küçükçekmece. Among the households that were reached, some households did not speak Turkish, had no eligible women, or could not participate for other reasons. In total, 8,100 women (4,164 women in Bağcılar and 3,936 women in Küçükçekmece) were asked to participate in the survey, and 4,122 (50.9 %) completed the survey, 3,270 (40.4 %) were not available after three attempts, and 606 (7.5 %) refused to participate.

Before the start of the study, the field company made many visits to the study areas and found few women who could only speak Kurdish; thus, the decision was made to exclude Kurdish language from the survey. Female enumerators, all employed by a local field company who carried out the field work, approached women in their homes, introduced themselves, informed women they were conducting a study about reproductive health, and screened women for eligibility. All married women between the ages of 15–44 who were usual residents of the households in the study communities, could consent to participation, and could communicate in Turkish were eligible for the study. Due to the topic of the study and the sensitive nature of our survey questions, the study focused only on married women. If more than one eligible woman lived in a household, we randomly selected one to participate using a randomization mechanism through our web-based data collection application. In Bağcılar, 18 households had more than one eligible woman, and in Küçükçekmece, 13 households had more than one eligible woman.

Women were provided details about the study, including the nature of the study, research objectives, benefits and risks, contact information for study investigators, and how their privacy would be maintained. The informed consent script was read aloud to women, including a portion on women's rights to refuse to participate, not answer any question(s), or withdraw from the study. Enumerators asked participants to provide oral consent to take part in the study. Women were provided small kitchen items, amounting to $5 USD, as compensation for interviews.

Enumerators interviewed women using hand-held tablets. Interviews were conducted in locations that provided visual and audio privacy. Only the enumerator and the respondent were present during the interview. The survey included questions about women's sociodemographic background and reproductive and contraceptive history. At the end of the survey, women were given the opportunity to make comments and ask questions.

2.2 Measures

Our primary outcome was the type of contraceptive method women reported using (0 = no method, 1 = traditional method, 2 = modern method). We asked women, "Are you or your husband/partner currently doing something or using any method to delay or avoid getting pregnant?" If yes, then we asked women to list which methods women or their husbands/partners were using. We classified barrier methods (i.e., male condoms, female condoms, diaphragms/sponges, spermicides), hormonal methods (i.e., pills, injectables, emergency contraception), and long-acting methods (i.e., implants, IUDs, and sterilization) as modern contraceptive methods. We classified withdrawal, calendar method/standard days/rhythm method, lactational amenorrhea method (LAM), and other folk methods as traditional or other methods. Finally, women not using any strategy to avoid pregnancy were classified as not using a method.

Our primary independent variables were ethnicity, region of birth, and time residing in one's neighborhood. Ethnicity was measured with one question asking women to self-report their ethnic identity. We created three ethnic categories: Turkish, Kurdish, or Other. The "other" category included women who identified as no ethnicity (n = 318), Arabic (n = 41), and other minority groups (i.e., Georgian, Kyrgyz, Turkmen, Azerbaijanis, Syrian, and Zaza; n = 8). Region of birth was a five-level categorical variable indicating the region of Turkey where the woman was born. These regions were based on the TDHS classifications (1 = West, 2 = South, 3 = Central, 4 = North, 5 = East). Women born outside of Turkey were excluded from the analysis. Finally, we created a four-level categorical variable indicating the length of time the woman resided in her current neighborhood (1 = less than 1 year, 2 = 1–5 years, 3 = 5–10 years, 4 = more than 10 years).

2.3 Analytical Strategy

To limit the sample to women who were at risk for unintended pregnancy, we excluded pregnant women (n = 312) and women who desired to become pregnant within the next 2 years (n = 437). Thus, the analysis included 3,038 women who were not pregnant or trying to become pregnant and with complete information. In descriptive analyses, we examined participant characteristics, ethnicity, and contraceptive method use. We used chi-square tests to assess differences across ethnic groups and contraceptive method use.

In the multivariate analysis, we implemented multinomial logit regression analyses to assess the relationship between contraceptive method use and ethnicity, region of birth, and time in neighborhood, adjusting for control variables. Then, we used the same approach to conduct subgroup analyses stratifying by ethnic group. We limited the subgroup analysis to Turkish and Kurdish ethnic identities as these are the two major ethnic groups in the region. Data were weighted to account for the survey's sampling design. In the adjusted models, we controlled for women's age, wealth, education, number of living children, employment, and district of residence in the models. We used Stata version 16 for analyses.

3 Results

The majority of participants identified as Turkish (59.4 %); 33.1 % identified as Kurdish and 7.4 % identified as another ethnic group (Tab. 6.1). Most participants were born in either the Eastern or Western regions (48.2 % and 30.7 %, respectively). Among women who identified as Turkish, 44.1 % were born in the Western region. Among women who identified as Kurdish, 90.6 % were born in the Eastern region. Almost half (48.9 %) of participants had lived in their neighborhood for more than 10 years. Larger proportions of Kurdish women had lived in their neighborhoods for 10 or less years, compared to women who identified as Turkish and another ethnic group. Most participants were aged 30 years or older (76.1 %) and half had completed primary school. Approximately 95 % of women were unemployed and, on average, women had 2.7 living children. Self-reported ethnicity was significantly associated with all demographic variables.

Tab. 6.1: Selected background characteristics of participants by ethnicity, among married women aged 15–44 years, Istanbul, Turkey

Characteristics		Ethnicity			
	Total (N = 3,038)	**Turkish (n = 1,805)**	**Kurdish (n = 1,007)**	**Other (n = 226)**	***P* value X^2**
Region					
West	30.7	44.1	8.0	24.3	0.000
South	2.7	3.3	1.2	4.4	
Central	8.7	12.9	0.2	13.7	
North	9.7	15.2	0.0	8.9	
East	48.2	24.5	90.6	48.7	
Time in neighborhood (in years)					
<1	2.5	2.3	2.8	2.7	0.000
1–5	18.0	17.7	19.0	16.4	
5–10	30.6	28.8	36.0	21.2	
>10	48.9	51.2	42.3	59.7	
Age					
16–19	0.3	0.4	0.2	0.0	0.001
20–24	6.1	5.9	6.5	6.2	
25–29	17.5	15.5	21.1	17.7	
30–34	22.3	21.2	23.6	24.8	
35–39	25.4	25.3	25.3	26.6	
40–44	28.4	31.8	23.3	24.8	
Wealth					
Poorest	14.4	11.3	19.9	15.0	0.000
Poorer	26.8	25.0	31.3	21.7	
Middle	22.7	23.9	19.1	29.7	
Richer	23.3	25.3	18.0	31.9	
Richest	12.7	14.6	11.8	1.8	
Education					
None / Primary incomplete	22.0	12.6	38.5	23.0	0.000
Primary school	50.0	53.5	44.6	46.9	
Secondary school	15.2	17.7	10.6	15.5	
High school and higher	12.8	16.3	6.3	14.6	
No. of living children	2.7 (1.3)[a]	2.5 (1.1)[a]	3.2 (1.5)[a]	2.7 (1.1)[a]	0.000

Tab. 6.1: Continued

Characteristics	Total (N = 3,038)	Ethnicity Turkish (n = 1,805)	Kurdish (n = 1,007)	Other (n = 226)	*P* value X^2
Work status					
Unemployed	95.4	95.0	96.8	92.0	0.000
Employed	4.6	5.0	3.2	8.0	
District					
Küçükçekmece	49.7	43.6	66.9	21.2	0.000
Bağcılar	50.3	56.4	33.1	78.8	

Note: all numbers are percentages unless otherwise stated
[a] Mean (SD)

Approximately 46 % of women were using a modern contraceptive method; 39.2 % of women were using a traditional method and 14.6 % were not using a contraceptive method (Tab. 6.2). Contraceptive method use was significantly associated with ethnicity, region of birth, and time in neighborhood. Larger proportions of Turkish women did not use a method (64.3 %), compared to traditional (58.4 %) or modern methods (58.7 %). In contrast, larger proportions of Kurdish women used modern methods (34.7 %) or traditional methods (32.7 %) than no method (29.6 %).

Tab. 6.2: Percent of women using each category of family planning method

Characteristics	No method[a] (n = 443)	Traditional method[b] (n = 1,190)	Modern method[c] (n = 1,405)	*P* value T^2
All women	14.6	39.2	46.3	-
Ethnicity				
Turkish	64.3	58.4	58.7	0.000
Kurdish	29.6	32.7	34.7	
Other	6.1	8.9	6.6	
Region				
West	39.3	26.6	31.5	0.000
South	3.4	2.0	3.1	
Central	8.1	8.9	8.8	
North	8.4	10.3	9.5	
East	40.9	52.2	47.2	

(Continued)

Tab. 6.2: Continued

Characteristics	No method[a] (n = 443)	Traditional method[b] (n = 1,190)	Modern method[c] (n = 1,405)	*P* value T^2
Time in neighborhood (in years)				
<1	3.4	2.6	2.1	0.000
1–5	24.2	18.0	16.1	
5–10	25.5	32.7	30.5	
>10	47.0	46.7	51.3	
Age				
16–19	1.1	0.2	0.1	0.000
20–24	10.4	6.6	4.3	
25–29	14.9	19.3	16.7	
30–34	17.4	23.3	22.9	
35–39	18.7	24.0	28.7	
40–44	37.5	26.6	27.2	
Wealth				
Poorest	16.0	13.5	14.7	0.029
Poorer	23.0	28.0	27.1	
Middle	26.2	23.4	21.1	
Richer	21.4	24.3	23.1	
Richest	13.3	10.8	14.1	
Education				
None / Primary incomplete	25.5	21.3	21.4	0.054
Primary school	47.7	52.1	49.0	
Secondary school	12.9	15.0	16.1	
High school and higher	13.8	11.6	13.6	
No. of living children	2.3 (1.4)[d]	2.6 (1.2)[d]	2.9 (1.3)[d]	0.000
Work status				
Unemployed	92.1	96.6	95.4	0.000
Employed	7.9	3.4	4.6	
District				
Küçükçekmece	40.2	55.0	48.2	0.000
Bağcılar	59.8	45.0	51.8	

[a] Includes women reporting no pregnancy prevention measures; [b] Withdrawal, standard days/calendar method/rhythm method, lactational amenorrhea method, and other traditional methods; [c] Condoms, oral contraceptives, injectables, implants, IUDs, sterilization, and other modern methods; [d] Mean (SD)

Tab. 6.3: Adjusted relative risk ratios (RRR) between sociodemographic variables and contraceptive use

	Traditional method versus no method		**Modern method versus no method**	
Characteristics	**RRR**	**95 % CI**	**RRR**	**95 % CI**
Ethnicity (ref: Turkish)				
Kurdish	0.69*	0.50, 0.96	0.94	0.68, 1.29
Other	1.60	0.99, 2.55	1.16	0.72, 1.87
Region (ref: West)				
South	0.75	0.37, 1.51	0.92	0.48, 1.76
Central	1.28**	1.15, 2.76	1.44	0.94, 2.21
North	2.00**	1.31, 3.07	1.54*	1.01, 2.35
East	2.03**	1.47, 2.80	1.30	0.94, 1.78
Time in neighborhood (in years) (ref: > 10)				
<1	0.70	0.35, 1.38	0.59	0.30, 1.16
1–5	0.71*	0.51, 0.98	0.65*	0.47, 0.91
5–10	1.08	0.81, 1.44	0.98	0.74, 1.29
Age (ref: 40–44)				
16–19	0.46	0.08, 2.58	0.53	0.10, 2.94
20–24	1.61	0.97, 2.66	1.21	0.73, 2.02
25–29	2.64**	1.78, 3.91	2.48**	1.68, 3.65
30–34	2.37**	1.68, 3.33	2.39**	1.71, 3.34
35–39	2.01**	1.46, 2.76	2.35**	1.72, 3.21
Wealth (ref: Poorest)				
Poorer	1.34	0.93, 1.95	1.18	0.82, 1.70
Middle	1.08	0.74, 1.57	0.88	0.61, 1.27
Richer	1.32	0.89, 1.95	1.11	0.76, 1.63
Richest	1.06	0.68, 1.66	1.17	0.76, 1.80
Education (ref: None / Primary incomplete)				
Primary school	1.65**	1.22, 2.24	1.70**	1.26, 2.30
Secondary school	2.05**	1.35, 3.13	2.76**	1.82, 4.18
High school and higher	1.51	0.98, 2.33	2.34**	1.53, 3.57
No. of living children	1.31**	1.17, 1.47	1.58**	1.42, 1.77
Employed	0.45**	0.28, 0.73	0.63*	0.40, 0.98
Lives in Bağcılar district	0.49**	0.34, 0.63	0.69**	0.55, 0.88

* $p < 0.05$, ** $p < 0.01$

Tab. 6.4: Adjusted relative risk ratios (RRR) of contraceptive use by region of birth and time of residing in neighborhood, stratified by ethnicity

		Traditional method versus no method		Modern method versus no method	
Ethnicity		**RRR**	**95 % CI**	**RRR**	**95 % CI**
Turkish	*Region (ref: West)*				
(n = 1,805)	South	0.69	0.30, 1.58	0.98	0.47, 2.09
	Central	1.89**	1.17, 3.06	1.58	0.99, 2.53
	North	2.06**	1.31, 3.22	1.49	0.96, 2.32
	East	2.06**	1.39, 3.05	1.17	0.79, 1.74
	Time in neighborhood (in years) (ref: >10)				
	<1	0.8437	0.35, 2.02	074	0.31, 1.77
	1–5	1.125	0.72, 1.76	0.88	0.57, 1.37
	5–10	1.382	0.96, 2.00	1.05	0.73, 1.52
Kurdish	*Region (ref: West)*				
(n = 1,007)	South	0.54	0.12, 2.48	0.14*	0.02, 0.96
	Central	0.00	0.00, 0.00	0.36	0.02, 7.06
	East	1.64	0.78, 3.43	1.46	0.71, 2.99
	Time in neighborhood (in years) (ref: >10)				
	<1	0.55	0.16, 1.92	0.46	0.13, 1.61
	1–5	0.40**	0.22, 0.71	0.46**	0.26, 0.80
	5–10	0.81	0.49, 1.36	0.85	0.52, 1.42

* $p < 0.05$, ** $p < 0.01$

Notes: Models are adjusted for age, wealth, education, number of living children, work status, and district

In the multivariate regression analyses, some contraceptive method use differed by ethnicity, region of birth, and time in neighborhood (Tab. 6.3). Kurdish women were less likely than Turkish women to use traditional methods over no method (Relative risk ratio [RRR] 0.70; 95 % CI 0.50, 0.96). However, there were no significant differences between Kurdish and Turkish women and use of modern methods. Women of other ethnic identities were similar in their use of traditional and modern methods to Turkish women.

Traditional method use varied by region of birth. In general, women born in regions farther away from Istanbul (located in the West region) were significantly more at risk of using traditional methods (e.g., RRR_{east} 2.02; 95 % CI 1.46,

2.79) than no method. Only women born in the North region were significantly more at risk of using modern methods, compared to no method, than women born in the West region (RRR 1.55; 95 % CI 1.01, 2.35). Women residing in their neighborhood 1–5 years were at less risk of using a traditional method (RRR 0.79; 95 % CI 0.50, 098) and modern method (RRR 0.65; 95 % CI 0.47, 0.91) rather than no method, compared to women who lived in the neighborhood for more than 10 years. However, women who lived in their neighborhood less than 1 year or 5–10 years were not different in their contraceptive behaviors from women who were living in their neighborhood for more than 10 years.

In the subgroup analyses, many differences emerged between Turkish and Kurdish women (Tab. 6.4). For Turkish women, time living in their neighborhood was not associated with use of traditional or modern methods. Additionally, region of birth was not significantly associated with modern contraceptive use. However, regarding traditional method use, women who were born in regions farther away from the West region had a greater risk of using traditional methods (RRR_{North} 2.06; 95 % CI 1.31, 3.22).

For Kurdish women, living in their neighborhood for 1–5 years was associated with reduced risk of using traditional (RRR 0.40; 95 % CI 0.22, 0.71) or modern methods (RRR 0.46; 95 % CI 0.26, 0.80) rather than for more than 10 years, compared to no method. In contrast to Turkish women, region of birth was not associated with traditional method versus no method use; while Kurdish women who were born in the South region were at less risk of using a modern method versus no method (RRR 0.14; 95 % CI 0.02, 0.96), compared to Kurdish women born in the West region.

4 Discussion

In our study, we did not find an association between self-reported ethnicity and use of modern contraceptive methods in two districts of urban Istanbul. Women who identified as Kurdish were less likely to use traditional methods than women who identified as Turkish; however, we hypothesize that this difference may be due to other factors, namely assimilation to other cultures measured with a proxy, time living in one's neighborhood. Regional variations in contraceptive use were concentrated only among Turkish women (i.e., Turkish women born in regions farther from the Western region were more likely to use traditional methods) and for traditional methods, rather than modern methods; however, there was less variation in region of birth for Kurdish women.

Our study, to our knowledge, is the first to examine the relationship between self-reported ethnic identity and contraceptive use in Turkey. In general, there is a limited literature about self-identifying Kurdish women's family planning behaviors. We limited our sample to Turkish-peaking women, and thus, we excluded women who speak Kurdish only. It is possible that among women who speak Turkish (the official language of Turkey), ethnic identity makes no difference, as these women can all reasonably access health services and information which are typically provided in Turkish. If we had also included women who speak only Kurdish, it is possible that we may have found differences between Turkish and Kurdish speaking women. Women who speak only Kurdish may be likely to experience more barriers to accessing family planning services, as compared to women who speak both Kurdish and Turkish.

Previous studies are conflicting as to whether Kurdish-speaking women and couples are more likely to use traditional methods and/or less likely to use modern methods. A study that assessed the relationship between cultural characteristics and use of withdrawal in Turkey found that couples who both spoke only Kurdish were more likely than couples who both spoke only Turkish to use withdrawal. However, there were no differences between couples who spoke only Turkish and couples that spoke both languages (Ergöçmen et al., 2004). A study using the husband's module from the 1998 TDHS found that there were no significant differences between men who spoke Turkish and men who spoke other languages in use of withdrawal (Kulczycki, 2004). Other studies using the 2013 TDHS provide evidence that Kurdish-peaking women are less likely to use modern contraception (Erman & Behrman, 2019; Karaoğlan & Saraçoğlu, 2018). Some of these studies did not focus on women only or the use of modern methods, and no studies asked participants to self-report ethnic identity; however, the studies suggest that language, one aspect of ethnic identity, may be meaningful in explaining disparities in family planning use in Turkey.

We found some evidence of regional variation (a proxy for ethnicity and sociocultural norms) in traditional method use. Turkey is the only country, outside of countries in Africa, with a method-mix skewed towards traditional methods (Bertrand et al., 2000), and withdrawal in particular. There is documented regional variation in traditional method use in Turkey. The 2018 TDHS reported that use of withdrawal was higher in the Northern (25.0 %), Eastern (22.5.%), and Central (20.9 %) regions than the Southern (17.7 %) and Western (19.6 %) regions (Hacettepe University Institute of Population Studies, 2019). It may be that women who were born in regions where use of withdrawal is common and a part of regional traditional are more likely to be familiar with and/or prefer the method. Interestingly, during the 1990s, use of withdrawal was highest in the Western and Eastern region, 28 % and 31 %, respectively, and lowest in the Eastern (14.4 %) region (Hacettepe University Institute of Population Studies,

1999). Kulczycki (2004) found that men from the Eastern and Central regions were significantly less likely to use withdrawal using the 1998 TDHS and speculated that the practice of withdrawal originated in Istanbul, and while it had slowly dispersed to other parts of the country, use was traditionally concentrated in Istanbul. Today, it may be that adoption of modern methods is now concentrated in Istanbul and may follow similar patterns of regional adoption in the future.

Our study is not without limitations. We are unable to generalize beyond the study sample. However, the survey was conducted in a large sample of married, reproductive age women who fit the profile of many other women in urban areas of developing countries. Further, we did not achieve a high response rate (51 %), compared to nationally representative surveys, such as the 2018 TDHS (81 %). The primary reason for non-response in our survey was failure to contact women at home after several repeated attempts (40.4 % of women in our survey were unreachable), similar to DHS. Regardless, we achieved our target sample size that was needed to detect a five-percentage point difference in the modern contraceptive prevalence rate between the intervention and comparison groups (the primary aim of the parent study).

Our study provides insight into ethnic and regional variations in contraceptive method use in Turkey. While previous reports have documented systematic barriers in health service utilization for ethnic minority populations (namely, Kurdish individuals), we did not find disparities in family planning use by self-reported ethnic identity. Future studies should consider how language also shapes family planning adoption and discontinuation. Further, regional variations in traditional method use deserve more attention.

References

Armstrong, K., Ravenell, K. L., McMurphy, S., & Putt, M. (2007). Racial/ethnic differences in physician distrust in the United States. *American Journal of Public Health*, *97*(7), 1283–1289. https://doi.org/10.2105/AJPH.2005.080762

Arslan, S. (2015). *Language policy in Turkey and its effect on the Kurdish language* [Master's Theses, Western Michigan University]. https://scholarworks.wmich.edu/masters_theses/620

Bearak, J., Popinchalk, A., Ganatra, B., Moller, A. B., Tunçalp, Ö., Beavin, C., Kwok, L., & Alkema, L. (2020). Unintended pregnancy and abortion by income, region, and the legal status of abortion: Estimates from a comprehensive model for 1990–2019. *The Lancet Global Health*, 8, e1152–e1161. https://doi.org/10.1016/S2214-109X(20)30315-6

Becker, D., & Tsui, A. O. (2008). Reproductive health service preferences and perceptions of quality among low-income women: Racial, ethnic, and language group differences. *Perspectives on Sexual and Reproductive Health*, *40*(4), 202–211. https://doi.org/10.1363/4020208

Bellizzi, S., Mannava, P., Nagai, M., & Sobel, H. L. (2020). Reasons for discontinuation of contraception among women with a current unintended pregnancy in 36 low and middle- income countries. *Contraception*, *101*(1), 26–33. https://doi.org/10.1016/j.contraception.2019.09.006

Bertrand, J., Rice, J., Sullican, T. M., & James, S. (2000). Skewed method mix: A measure of quality in family planning programs. *Measure evaluation.* file:///C:/Users/huber/AppData/Local/Temp/wp-00- 23.pdf

Brockerhoff, M., & Hewett, P. (2000). Inequality of child mortality among ethnic groups in sub- Saharan Africa. *Bulletin of the World Health Organization*, *78*(1), 30–41.

Central Intelligence Agency. (2020, August 5). *The World Factbook: Turkey. The World Factbook*. https://www.cia.gov/library/publications/the-world-factbook/geos/tu.html

De Broe, S., Hinde, A., Matthews, Z., & Padmadas, S. S. (2005). Diversity in family planning use among ethnic groups in Guatemala. *Journal of Biosocial Science*, *37*(3), 301–317. https://doi.org/10.1017/S0021932004006650

Dehlendorf, C., Foster, D. G., de Bocanegra, H. T., Brindis, C., Bradsberry, M., & Darney, P. (2011). Race, ethnicity and differences in contraception among low-income women: Methods received by family PACT clients, California, 2001–2007. *Perspectives on Sexual and Reproductive Health, 43*(3), 181–187. https://doi.org/10.1363/4318111

Dehlendorf, C., Park, S. Y., Emeremni, C. A., Comer, D., Vincett, K., & Borrero, S. (2014). Racial/ethnic disparities in contraceptive use: Variation by age and women's reproductive experiences. *American Journal of Obstetrics and Gynecology*, *210*(6), 526.e1–526.e9. https://doi.org/10.1016/j.ajog.2014.01.037

Ergöçmen, B. A., Koç, I., Senlet, P., Yiğit, E. K., & Roman, E. (2004). A closer look at traditional contraceptive use in Turkey. *The European Journal of Contraception & Reproductive Health Care*, *9*(4), 221–244. https://doi.org/10.1080/13625180400017768

Erman, J., & Behrman, J. (2019). *Internal migration and contraceptive use in Turkey.* Population Association of America. http://paa2019.populationassociation.org/uploads/192189

European Counrt of Human Rights. (2015). *Annual Report 2014 of the European Court of Human Rights, Council of Europe.* Registry of the European Counrt of Human Rights. https://echr.coe.int/Documents/Annual_Report_2014_ENG.pdf

Grady, C. D., Dehlendorf, C., Cohen, E. D., Schwarz, E. B., & Borrero, S. (2015). Racial and ethnic differences in contraceptive use among women who desire no future children, 2006–2010 National Survey of Family Growth. *Contraception*, *92*(1), 62–70. https://doi.org/10.1016/j.contraception.2015.03.017

Guendelman, S., Denny, C., Mauldon, J., & Chetkovich, C. (2000). Perceptions of hormonal contraceptive safety and side effects among low-income Latina and non-Latina women. *Maternal and Child Health Journal*, *4*(4), 233–239. https://doi.org/10.1023/a:1026643621387

Hacettepe University Institute of Population Studies. (1999). *Turkish Demographic and Health Survey, 1998*. Hacettepe University. https://dhsprogram.com/pubs/pdf/FR108/FR108.pdf

Hacettepe University Institute of Population Studies. (2019). *2018 Turkey Demographic and Health Survey.*

Human Rights Watch. (2006). *Unjust, restrictive, and inconsistent: The impact of Turkey's compensation law with respect to internally displaced people* (No. 1; pp. 1–39). Human Rights Watch. https://www.hrw.org/legacy/backgrounder/eca/turkey1206/turkey1206web.pdf

Karaoğlan, D., & Saraçoğlu, D. S. (2018). *Women's education, employment status and the choice of birth control method: An investigation for the case of Turkey* (ERC Working Paper No. 1803). ERC – Economic Research Center, Middle East Technical University.

Kennedy, B. R., Mathis, C. C., & Woods, A. K. (2007). African Americans and their distrust of the health care system: Healthcare for diverse populations. *Journal of Cultural Diversity*, *14*(2), *56–60.*

Kulczycki, A. (2004). The determinants of withdrawal use in Turkey: A husband's imposition or a woman's choice? *Social Science & Medicine*, *59*(5), 1019–1033. https://doi.org/10.1016/j.socscimed.2003.12.014

McNamee, C. B. (2009). Wanted and unwanted fertility in Bolivia: Does ethnicity matter? *International Perspectives on Sexual and Reproductive Health*, *35*(4), 166–175. https://doi.org/10.1363/ipsrh.35.166.09

Mishra, M. (2010). Ethnic disparities in contraceptive use and its impact on family planning program in Nepal. *Journal of Family and Reproductive Health*, *43*(3), 121–128.

Saatçi, E., & Akpınar, E. (2007). Assessing poverty and related factors in Turkey. *Croatian Medical Journal*, *48*, 628–635.

Sangi-Haghpeykar, H., Ali, N., Posner, S., & Poindexter, A. N. (2006). Disparities in contraceptive knowledge, attitude and use between Hispanic and non-Hispanic whites. *Contraception*, *74*(2), 125–132. https://doi.org/10.1016/j.contraception.2006.02.010

Sulaivany, K. (2019, December 8). Language barrier leads to inequality for Kurds in accessing healthcare in Turkey. *Kurdistan 24*. https://www.kurdistan24.net/en/news/deda867f-491f-403c-8146-9b2458f4c328

Yüceşahin, M. M., & Özgür, E. M. (2008). Regional fertility differences in Turkey: Persistent high fertility in the southeast. *Population, Space and Place*, *14*(2), 135–158. https://doi.org/10.1002/psp.480

BAHAR AYÇA OKÇUOĞLU, SARAH HUBER-KRUM

7 Associations between Women's Empowerment, Conservatism and Contraceptive Trends

Abstract: Women's fertility planning and contraceptive decision-making cannot be adequately understood by focusing only on the historical, political and economic contexts. Women's attitudes and values may be important determinants of their reproductive health behaviors, as values affect a variety of aspects of everyday life in Turkey and elsewhere. Accordingly, women's family planning and contraceptive method preferences may be, in part, driven by their attitudes towards conservatism, religiosity, decision-making power (empowerment), and their autonomy. How might these aspects, controlling for other confounding factors, affect women's preferences on contraceptive usage and method choice? This chapter aims to explain the relationship between these four aspects and contraceptive use, including method mix, from a large study conducted in Istanbul.

Keywords: Reproductive health behaviors, religiosity, women's empowerment, contraceptive trends, conservatism.

1 Introduction

Women's fertility planning and contraceptive decision-making cannot be adequately understood by focusing only on the historical, political, and economic contexts alone. Women's attitudes and values may be important determinants of their reproductive health behaviors, as beliefs affect a variety of aspects of health decision-making. Previous studies acknowledge the influence of religion and culture on sexual and reproductive behavior (Arousell & Carlbom, 2016; Moreau et al., 2013; Rostosky et al., 2004). Accordingly, women's family planning and contraceptive method preferences may be, in part, driven by their attitudes towards conservatism, religiosity, empowerment, and their autonomy. How might these aspects, controlling for other confounding factors, affect women's preferences on contraceptive usage and method choice? This chapter aims to examine the relationship between these four aspects and contraceptive use, including method mix, by utilizing cross-sectional data from a large study conducted in Istanbul, Turkey.

1.1 Women's Empowerment and Values on Contraceptive Decision-Making

Women's empowerment, defined as "process by which those who have been denied the ability to make strategic life choices acquire such an ability" is increasingly considered a key factor in women's family planning and reproductive health decisions (Kabeer, 1999, p. 2). It may be that as women are more able to make strategic life choices (i.e., as they become empowered), they might also develop a preference to plan for their futures, decide on their life roles such as getting married or having children, plan for their pregnancies and use family planning methods. Income and education are factors for women to feel empowered and assess the impact of their actions and the future outcomes (Korteweg, 2008). "Women's access to better socio-economic resources empowers them towards organizing and taking decisions about their own lives, as well as on birth control choices" (Cindoğlu et al., 2008, p. 416). However, the measurement of women's empowerment is difficult because it is multidimensional. The same is true for religiosity, conservatism, and autonomy.

Women's lack of power is assumed to affect their decisions about family planning, and their lack of decision-making power may restrict the use of modern contraceptives (Do & Kurimoto, 2012). Women's economic dependency on their partner - a dimension of empowerment and autonomous decision-making - may also influence contraceptive decision-making and method choices (Sirkeci & Cindoğlu, 2012). Findings from Demographic and Health Surveys (DHS) conducted between 2006 and 2008 in Namibia, Zambia, Ghana, and Uganda with women aged 15–49 suggest positive associations between empowerment and method use in all countries (Do & Kurimoto, 2012). A study carried out in Oman also suggests that empowered women are more likely to use contraception (Al Riyami et al., 2004). Women's autonomy – another aspect of women's empowerment – may also influence family planning decisions. A study conducted in Eritrea found a positive relationship between women's autonomy and reproductive preferences (Woldemicael, 2009). Findings from a study conducted in Bangladesh also indicated that household decision-making autonomy is significantly associated with the current use of modern contraception (Rahman et al., 2014).

Religion, religiosity, and conservatism may also influence women's and couple's contraceptive decisions. A study using data from 22 countries found that Muslim women may lack comprehensive knowledge about sexual and reproductive health, which affects their access to the services (Alomair et al., 2020). There are also barriers like misconceptions and negative attitudes towards family planning, such as limiting the number of children in respect of their religious values. The study also claims that husbands' and families' opposition affect women's contraceptive use significantly (Alomair et al., 2020). A study carried out in Istanbul, Turkey found that cultural and religious norms were not barriers to contraceptive use, but did influence the selection a method (Cebeci et al., 2004). In Kocaeli, Turkey, women's contraceptive behavior may be influenced by their husbands' attitudes and increasing the education level of women significantly increased contraceptive use (Vural et al., 1999). A qualitative study involving focus group discussions and in-depth interviews with two predominant Muslim communities in Kenya proposes that there are various interpretations of Islamic teaching, whether Islam allows family planning method use or not (Abdi et al., 2020).

With a majority of Muslim population, religious values have always been an influential factor in people's everyday lives in Turkey, including contraception. "Religion was identified as a key variable determining contraceptive method and withdrawal was perceived to be a suitable modality according to religion in earlier studies in Turkey, which reported that local religious leaders favoured this 'natural and harmless' method which was also 'encouraged by the Prophet'" (Cindoğlu et al., 2008, p. 413). This might partially explain the high prevalence of withdrawal use among women in Turkey. The 2018 Turkey DHS reported contraceptive knowledge and usage in a specific time period for Turkey. The knowledge on contraceptive methods is high in Turkey: 99 % of all women and 99 % of married women have heard about a contraceptive method. Overall, 70 % of currently married women use a method of family planning. The most commonly used method is withdrawal (20 %), followed by male condom (19 %), IUD (14 %), and sterilization (10 %). The percentage of currently married women aged 15–49 currently using any contraceptive method decreased from 74 % in 2013 to 70 % in 2018 (Hacettepe University Institute of Population Studies, 2019), 2019).

Considering the literature on women's values on contraceptive decision-making and background information on Turkey, this study aims to understand how women's attitudes towards conservatism, religiosity, empowerment, and autonomy might affect their preferences on contraceptive usage and method choice. The following sections will analyze these factors and their effects from a large study conducted in Istanbul.

2 Methods

2.1 Setting and Study Design

We conducted a cross-sectional, household survey with married women of reproductive age (16–44) in two districts of Istanbul, Bağcılar and Küçükçekmece, between March and June 2018. This survey was part of the Willows Study, an impact evaluation of the Willow's International Reproductive Health Program. We used GIS mapping to demarcate boundaries for the site where intervention was planned following the survey (Bağcılar) and the comparison site (Küçükçekmece). Using the National Statistics Institute (TUIK) address list, we randomly sampled streets in each site to be surveyed. For streets with more than 100 households in Bağcılar or more than 200 households in Küçükçekmece, households were randomly sampled, and eligible women were interviewed. In total, 4,224 women participated in the survey.

2.2 Measures

Our analysis included four outcomes. Our first outcome of interest was whether women were using any method of family planning or not (coded binary). Next, we constructed a variable to capture whether women were using a modern method (i.e., condoms, pills, injections, implants, IUDs, emergency contraception, sterilization, and other modern methods) versus other family planning methods (i.e., withdrawal, standard days/calendar, lactational amenorrhea, and other folk or traditional methods). Our third outcome was a four-level categorical variable measuring the type of modern method a woman was using (1 = sterilization, 2 = IUD, 3 = condom, 4 = other modern method). We focused on these methods as they are the most commonly used modern methods among women in the region.

Our primary explanatory variables included: conservative values, empowerment, religiosity, and autonomy. The conservative values, empowerment, and autonomy variables were created using factor analysis. Religiosity was measured with one question asking women how important religion is in women's lives (scale from 1 to 10, with 10 being the most important). The conservative values scale consisted of six different statements: (1) "My husband's family have right to take decisions on family matters"; (2) "Women should be virgin when they get married"; (3) "A woman has to have children in order to be fulfilled"; (4) "A woman can have a child as a single parent, when she doesn't want to have a stable relationship with a man"; (5) "It is a duty towards society to have children"; (6) "A woman who have a child should not divorce". Response options consisted of five options (1 = strongly agree with statement; 2 = Agree with statement; 3 = Neither agree nor disagree with statement; 4 = Disagree with statement; 5 = strongly disagree with statement). The autonomy scale consisted of five questions: (1) "Does he interfere your meetings with your woman friends?"; (2) "Does he restrict you to see your family?"; (3) "Does he insist to know always where you are?"; (4) "Does he have issues to trust you in financial matters?"; (5) "Does he accuse you of being disloyal?". Response options consisted of three options (1 = Often interferes; 2 = Sometimes interferes; 3 = Never interferes). The third scale, empowerment consisted of three different questions: (1) "Who usually decides how your (husband's) earnings will be used?"; (2) "Who usually makes decisions about health care for yourself?"; (3) "Who usually makes decisions about making major household purchases?". Response options recoded into two options (1 = Other and respondent; 2 = & Respondent and husband jointly).

Exact wording of all questions and response options for three scales can be found in Appendix 7.1. We controlled for women's age, education, and ethnicity in the adjusted models. All models include a fixed-effect for area of residence.

2.3 Analytical Strategy

Stata/IC 16.0 program was used for data management, coding, and analysis. We used univariate statistics to describe the prevalence of current use of family planning methods and women's background characteristics.

We used logistic and sequential logistic regressions to understand whether women's attitudes on the four exposures of interest were associated with (1) any use of family planning, (2) use of a modern method, (3) use of specific modern method, and (4) method mix. The first logistic regression presents the association between women's religiosity, conservative values, autonomy, and empowerment with use of any family planning method. The second logistic regression shows the four exposures of interest's association for current use of modern family planning among women using any family planning method. The sequential model presents the likelihood of women using any family planning method or not, and the likelihood of women using modern contraception among women using any family planning method.

3 Results and Discussion

3.1 Background Characteristics

Tab. 7.1: Selected background characteristics of women

	N	%
District		
Bağcılar	1,459	51.17
Küçükçekmece	1,529	48.83
Age categories		
16–19	8	0.27
20–24	197	6.59
25–29	549	18.37
30–34	700	23.43
35–39	773	25.87
40–44	761	25.47
Education		
None / Primary incomplete	473	15.87
Primary school	1,612	54.09
Secondary school	488	16.38
High school and higher	407	13.66
Ethnicity		
Turkish	1,735	58.24
Kurdish	981	32.93
Other	263	8.82

Table 7.1 describes the selected background characteristics of women included in the analysis. The number of women interviewed in selected districts were close to each other (Bağcılar = 1,459; Küçükçekmece = 1,529). Most of the women were aged between 35–39 years (25.87 %), and most women completed primary school (54.09 %). More than half of the sample identified as Turkish (58.24 %).

Tab. 7.2: Description of religiosity, conservative values, autonomy, and empowerment

	N	Mean	Std. Dev.	Range
Religiosity	2,983	9.72	0.96	1–10
Conservative values				1–5
(a) Husband's family's right	2,942	3.11	1.09	
(b) Virginity	2,950	1.99	0.85	
(c) Fulfillment with children	2,881	2.67	1.07	
(d) Woman as single parent	2,857	2.67	1.08	
(e) Having children as duty	2,920	3.12	1.18	
(f) Divorcement	2,795	3.17	1.27	
Autonomy				1–3
(a) Meeting with woman friends	2,979	2.72	0.50	
(b) To see family	2,979	2.87	0.36	
(c) Insists to know	2,979	2.56	0.64	
(d) Trust with financial matters	2,978	2.92	0.29	
(e) Accusation of being disloyal	2,976	2.94	0.23	
Empowerment				1–2
(a) Husband's earnings	2,971	1.91	0.28	
(b) Health care	2,978	1.96	0.19	
(c) Major household purchases	2,977	1.87	0.32	

The table (Tab. 7.2) for descriptive statistics shows results for women's selected characteristics and scales, who are included in the analysis. As mentioned above, the high score for religiosity question indicates high importance of religion in women's lives. This table shows that the mean of religiosity is close to 10 for women in this analysis. Means and standard deviations of three scales are shown in the table. It shows that women mostly disagree with the conservative value statements but agree with the statement on virginity. The autonomy scale response means shows that women mostly state that their husbands never interfere in their lives on various topics. Empowerment scale means shows that women and their husbands mostly decide jointly on earnings and expenses.

Tab. 7.3: Matrix of Pearson Correlation between primary independent variables

	(1)	(2)	(3)	(4)
(1) Religiosity	1.000			
(2) Cons. values	–0.151	1.000		
(3) Autonomy	0.128	0.064	1.000	
(4) Empowerment	-0.058	0.092	0.385	1.000

Table 7.3 highlights the correlations between religiosity, conservative values, autonomy, and empowerment. The correlations between autonomy and religiosity, conservative values, and empowerment were positive (Pearson correlation coefficients 0.128, 0.064, and 0.385, respectively) but weak. The correlation between empowerment and conservative values was also positive (Pearson correlation coefficient 0.092) and weak. However, the correlations between religiosity and conservative values (Pearson correlation coefficient −0.151) and empowerment (Pearson correlation coefficient −0.058) were negative and weak.

Tab. 7.4: Factor loadings (pattern matrix) and unique variances of constructs

	Factor 1	Factor 2	Factor 3	Uniqueness
Conservative values				
Husband's family's right	0.3861			0.8509
Virginity	0.5203			0.7293
Fulfillment with children	0.7325			0.4635
Woman as single parent	0.3143			0.9012
Having children as duty	0.7003			0.5096
Divorcement	0.7056			0.5022
Autonomy				
Meeting with woman friends		0.7250		0.4743
To see family		0.7610		0.4209
Insists to know		0.5419		0.7064
Trust with financial matters		0.7367		0.4572
Accusation of being disloyal		0.6917		0.5216
Empowerment				
Respondent's (husband's) earnings			0.6656	0.5569
Decisions about health care for the respondent			0.5470	0.7008
Decisions about making major household purchases			0.6569	0.5685

Factor loadings and unique variances of key constructs are presented in Tab. 7.4. Table 7.5 presents the percent distribution of women who were using any kind of family planning method. The most commonly used family planning methods were withdrawal (44.81 %), IUDs (20.82 %), male condoms (17.44 %) and female sterilization (9.54 %).

Tab. 7.5: Percent distribution of married women aged 15–49, by method of family planning using at time of survey

Contraceptive method	N	%
Female sterilization	285	9.54
IUD	622	20.82
Injectables	20	0.67
Pills	166	5.56
Male condoms	521	17.44
Female condoms	2	0.07
Emergency contraception	1	0.03
Standard days/Calendar method	6	0.20
Lactational Amenorrhea method	23	0.77
Withdrawal	1,339	44.81
Other method	3	0.10
Total	3,889	100.00

Table 7.6 presents the results for the logistic regression of use of any family planning method. Women's conservative values, autonomy, and empowerment were not associated with use of any family planning. Women who were more religious were 20 % more likely to use any method of family planning (OR: 1.20; 95 % CI: 1.12, 1.29). Women's age and education were also significantly associated with family planning use. As women's age increased, their likelihood of using any method of family planning decreased (OR: 0.89; 95 % CI: 0.85, 0.93). As compared to women who had no or incomplete primary education, women who had completed primary education were over 1.5 times more likely to use any method of family planning (OR: 1.70; 95 % CI: 1.35, 2.14). Similarly, women who had completed secondary school and high school or above had elevated odds of using any method of family planning (OR: 1.96; 95 % CI: 1.49, 2.59; OR: 1.85; 95 % CI: 1.39, 2.47, respectively). As women's number of living children increased, their likelihood of using any method of family planning increased (OR: 2.01; 95 % CI: 1.86, 2.17).

Tab. 7.6: Odds ratios (and 95 % confidence intervals) from logistic regression analyses examining associations between selected characteristics and current use of any family planning method

	OR	95 % CI
Religiosity	1.21**	1.12, 1.29
Cons. values	1.08	0.98, 1.18
Autonomy	0.93	0.85, 1.03
Empowerment	0.98	0.88, 1.10
District	0.98	0.83, 1.16
Age (measured in categories)	2.77**	1.91, 4.03
Age squared	0.89**	0.85, 0.93
Education (Ref: None / Primary incomplete)		
Primary school	1.70**	1.35, 2.14
Secondary school	1.96**	1.49, 2.59
High school and higher	1.85**	1.39, 2.47
Ethnicity (Ref: Turkish)		
Kurdish	0.84	0.69, 1.03
Other	1.05	0.78, 1.41
Number of living children	2.01**	1.86, 2.17

* $p < 0.05$, ** $p < 0.01$

Table 7.7 presents the logistic regression results for current use of modern family planning among women using any family planning method. Again, women's conservative values, autonomy, and empowerment were not associated with use of modern contraception among current family planning users. Women who were more religious were 10 % less likely to use modern contraception (OR: 0.90; 95 % CI: 0.82, 0.98). Women's district of residence, education, ethnicity, and number of living children were significantly associated with modern contraception. Women who were living in Bağcılar were 1.31 times more likely to use modern contraception (OR: 1.31; 95 % CI: 1.10, 1.55). As compared to women who had no or incomplete primary education, women who had completed high school or higher were 1.72 times more likely to use modern contraception (OR: 1.72; 95 % CI: 1.26, 2.35). As compared to Turkish women, women who identified as another ethnicity were 34 % less likely to use modern contraception (OR: 0.66; 95 % CI: 0.50, 0.88). As women's number of living children increased, their odds of using modern family planning increased (OR: 1.22; 95 % CI: 1.14, 1.31).

Tab. 7.7: Odds ratios (and 95 % confidence intervals) from logistic regression analyses examining associations between selected characteristics and current use of modern contraception

	OR	95 % CI
Religiosity	0.90*	0.82, 0.98
Cons. values	1.08	0.98, 1.18
Autonomy	0.95	0.86, 1.05
Empowerment	0.93	0.83, 1.04
District	1.31**	1.10, 1.55
Age categories	1.29	0.82, 2.01
Age square	0.97	0.92, 1.02
Education (Ref: None / Primary incomplete)		
Primary school	1.10	0.88, 1.38
Secondary school	1.31	0.98, 1.74
High school and higher	1.72**	1.26, 2.35
Ethnicity (Ref: Turkish)		
Kurdish	1.09	0.90, 1.33
Other	0.66**	0.50, 0.88
Number of living children	1.22**	1.14, 1.31

* $p < 0.05$, ** $p < 0.01$

Table 7.8 presents the results of the sequential logistic regression model. The first sequence presents the likelihood of women using any family planning method or not. In this panel, women's religiosity, age, education level, and number of living children were significantly associated with any family planning use. Religious women were 1.20 times more likely to use any family planning method (OR: 1.20; 95 % CI: 1.12, 1.29). As women's age increased, their likelihood of using any method of family planning decreased by 11 % (OR: 0.89; 95 % CI: 0.85, 0.93). As compared to women who had no or incomplete primary education, women who had completed primary school were 1.7 times more likely to use any method of family planning (OR: 1.70; 95 % CI: 1.35, 2.14). Similarly, women who had completed secondary or high school and above were more likely to use any method of family planning, compared to the same reference group (OR: 1.96; 95 % CI: 1.49, 2.59; OR: 1.85; 95 % CI: 1.39, 2.47, respectively). As women's number of living children increased, their likelihood of using any method of family planning increased (OR: 2.01; 95 % CI: 1.86, 2.17).

Tab. 7.8: Odds ratios (and 95 % confidence intervals) from sequential logistic regression analyses examining associations between selected characteristics

	OR	95 % CI
Use of any family planning method		
Religiosity	1.20**	1.12, 1.29
Cons. values	1.08	0.98, 1.18
Autonomy	0.93	0.85, 1.03
Empowerment	0.98	0.88, 1.10
District	0.98	0.83, 1.16
Age categories	2.77**	1.91, 4.03
Age square	0.89**	0.85, 0.93
Education (Ref: None / Primary incomplete)		
Primary school	1.70**	1.35, 2.14
Secondary school	1.96**	1.49, 2.59
High school and higher	1.85**	1.39, 2.47
Ethnicity (Ref: Turkish)		
Kurdish	0.84	0.69, 1.03
Other	1.05	0.78, 1.41
Number of living children	2.01**	0.00, 0.02
Use of modern contraception, among current users of any family planning method		
Religiosity	0.90*	0.82, 0.98
Cons. values	1.07	0.98, 1.18
Autonomy	0.95	0.87, 1.05
Empowerment	0.93	0.83, 1.04
District	1.31**	1.11, 1.55
Age categories	1.29	0.82, 2.01
Age square	0.97	0.92, 1.02
Education (Ref: None / Primary incomplete)		
Primary school	1.10	0.88, 1.38
Secondary school	1.31	0.98, 1.74
High school and higher	1.74**	1.28, 2.37
Ethnicity (Ref: Turkish)		
Kurdish	1.10	0.90, 1.33
Other	0.67**	0.51, 0.89
Number of living children	1.22**	1.13, 1.31

* p<0.05, ** p<0.01

The second sequence presents the likelihood of women using modern contraception among women using any family planning method. Religiosity, district, education, ethnicity, and number of living children were significantly associated with modern contraceptive use. Women who were more religious were 10 % less likely to use modern contraception (OR: 0.90; 95 % CI: 0.82, 0.98). Women who were living in Bağcılar were 1.31 times more likely to use modern contraception (OR: 1.31; 95 % CI: 1.11, 1.55). As compared to women who had no or incomplete primary education, women who had completed high school or higher were 1.74 times more likely to use modern contraception than traditional methods (OR: 1.74; 95 % CI: 1.28, 2.37). As compared to Turkish women, women who identified as another ethnicity were 33 % less likely to use modern contraception than traditional methods (OR: 0.67; 95 % CI: 0.51, 0.89). As women's number of living children increased, their likelihood of using a modern method of family planning instead of traditional methods increased by 1.2 times (OR: 1.22; 95 % CI: 1.13, 1.31).

4 Conclusion

This study aimed to understand how conservative values, religiosity, empowerment, and autonomy are related to contraceptive use and contraceptive method choices, by showing a cross-sectional data example from a large study conducted in Istanbul, Turkey. We found that religiosity is the most influential factor for contraceptive decision-making, along with women's educational level. The number of living children is also positively associated with the likelihood of using any family planning method. Contrary to the literature, our study shows that women's conservative values, autonomy, and empowerment were not associated with use of any family planning method, including the modern ones. In our analysis, as women mostly disagree with conservative statements, express that their husbands mostly do not interfere in their lives, and they jointly decide on earnings and expenses with their husbands, high levels of religiosity might be the only influential aspect on contraceptive use and method choice. Our results suggest that programs and policies regarding family planning should consider women's religiosity to increase the use of family planning methods, including modern contraception.

References

Abdi, B., Okal, J., Serour, G., & Temmerman, M. (2020). "Children are a blessing from God": A qualitative study exploring the socio-cultural factors influencing contraceptive use in two Muslim communities in Kenya. *Reproductive Health, 17*(1), 44.

Alomair, N., Alageel, S., Davies, N., & Bailey, J. V. (2020). Factors influencing sexual and reproductive health of Muslim women: A systematic review. *Reproductive Health, 17*(1), 33.

Al Riyami A., Afifi, M., & Mabry, R. M. (2004). Women's autonomy, education and employment in Oman and their influence on contraceptive use. *Reproductive Health Matters, 12*(23), 144–154.

Arousell, J., & Carlbom, A. (2016). Culture and religious beliefs in relation to reproductive health. *Best Practice & Research: Clinical Obstetrics & Gynaecology, 32*, 77–87.

Cebeci, D., Erbaydar, T., Kalaca, S., Harmancı, H., Çalı, S., & Karavuş, M. (2004). Resistance against contraception or medical contraceptive methods: A qualitative study on women and men in Istanbul. *The European Journal of Contraception and Reproductive Health Care, 9*, 94–101.

Cindoğlu, D., Sirkeci, I., & Sirkeci, F. (2008). Determinants of choosing withdrawal over modern contraceptive methods in Turkey. *The European Journal of Contraception and Reproductive Health Care, 13*(4), 412–421.

Do, M., & Kurimoto, N. (2012). Women's empowerment and choice of contraceptive methods in selected African countries. *International Perspectives on Sexual and Reproductive Health, 38*(1), 23–33. https://doi.org/10.1363/3802312

Hacettepe University Institute of Population Studies. (2019). *The 2018 Turkey Demographic and Health Survey (2018 TDHS).* Retrieved from https://dhsprogram.com/pubs/pdf/FR372/FR372.pdf.

Kabeer, N. (1999). *The conditions and consequences of choice: Reflections on the measurement of women's empowerment* (Discussion Paper No. 108). Geneva: United Nations Research Institute for Social Developments.

Korteweg, A. (2008). The Shari debate in Ontario: Gender, Islam, and representations of Muslim women's agency. *Gender and Society, 22*, 434–454.

Moreau, C., Trussell, J., & Bajos, N. (2013). Religiosity, religious affiliation, and patterns of sexual activity and contraceptive use in France. *The European Journal of Contraception & Reproductive Health Care, 18*(3), 168–80.

Rahman, M. M., Mostofa, M. G., & Hoque, M. A. (2014). Women's household decision-making autonomy and contraceptive behavior among Bangladeshi women. *Sexual & Reproductive Healthcare, 5*(1), 9–15.

Rostosky, S. S., Wilcox, B. L., Wright, M. L. C., & Randall, B. A. (2004). The impact of religiosity on adolescent sexual behavior: A review of the evidence. *Journal of Adolescent Research, 19*(6), 677–697.

Sirkeci, I., & Cindoğlu, D. (2012). Space, agency, and withdrawal: Birth control choices of women in Turkey. *Health Care for Women International, 33*, 614–630.

Vural, B., Vural, F., Diker, J., & Yucesoy, I. (1999). Factors affecting contraceptive use and behavior in Kocaeli, Turkey. *Advances in Contraception, 15(4)*, 325–336.

Woldemicael, G. (2009). Women's autonomy and reproductive preferences in Eritrea. *Journal of Biosocial Science, 41*(2), 161–181.

Appendix 7.1: Questions for conservative values, autonomy, and empowerment scales

		Response options
Conservative values	Now I would like to read some statements. Please tell me to what extent you agree or disagree	Strongly agree, Agree, Neither agree nor disagree, Disagree, Strongly disagree
(a) Husband's family's right	My husband's family have right to take decisions on family matters	
(b) Virginity	Women should be virgin when they get married	
(c) Fulfillment with children	A woman has to have children in order to be fulfilled	
(d) Woman as single parent	A woman can have a child as a single parent, when she doesn't want to have a stable relationship with a man	
(e) Having children as duty	It is a duty towards society to have children	
(f) Divorcement	A woman who have a child should not divorce	
Autonomy	Now I would like to read you some situations. Can you tell me how frequently you come through these with your husband/partner?	Often, Sometimes, Never
(a) Meeting with woman friends	Does he interfere your meetings with your woman friends?	
(b) To see family	Does he restrict you to see your family?	
c) Insists to know	Does he insist to know always where you are?	
(d) Trust with financial matters	Does he have issues to trust you in financial matters?	

(*Continued*)

Appendix 7.1: Continued

		Response options
(e) Accusation of being disloyal	Does he accuse you of being disloyal?	
Empowerment		Recoded as Other and Respondent & Respondent and husband jointly
(a) Who usually decides how your (husband's) earnings will be used?	Respondent, Husband, Respondent and husband jointly, Husband has no earnings, Other	
(b) Who usually makes decisions about health care for yourself?	Respondent, Husband, Respondent and husband jointly, Other male, Someone else	
(c) Who usually makes decisions about making major household purchases?	Respondent, Husband, Respondent and husband jointly, Other male, Someone else	

RYOKO SATO

8 Effect of Distance to, and Service Availability of, Health Facilities on Family Planning Use among Urban Turkish Women

Abstract: This chapter evaluates the effect of distance to a health facility, according to its service availability, on the family planning uptake among married Turkish women, while overcoming the challenges of data availability. We find that the effect of distance to a health facility on contraceptive use significantly differs according to FP availability at a health facility. Further, distance to a health facility that provides long-acting FP decreases the use of long-acting FP, while it has a substitute effect on the use of short-acting FP. When women face the accessibility barrier to a long-acting FP service, they modify their behaviors so that they shift from long-acting FP to short-acting FP, which is less effective.

Keywords: Fertility rate, effective contraceptive methods, long-acting FP, short-acting FP, logistic regression, female sterilization.

1 Introduction

High fertility rate around the world does not always reflect the desire and preference of reproduction among women. The unmet need for contraception has reached 21.6 % worldwide (Cahill et al., 2018), despite the increasing availability of effective contraceptive methods (Ali et al., 2018). Identifying barriers to the utilization of family planning (FP) is critical in reducing this unmet need.

One well-known demand-side barrier to health service utilization is access to a health facility. Extensive studies have examined the relationship between distance to a health facility and various health behaviors, and distance decay is often observed (Karra et al., 2017; Tegegne et al., 2018).

Some recent studies have evaluated the association between distance to a health facility and FP use. Many studies, however, found null effect of distance. For example, Yao et al. (2012) found that distance had no significant influence on using FP in Mozambique. Similarly, Heard et al. (2004) did not find any association between distance and modern contraceptive use in Malawi.

The insignificant distance effect found in existing studies might be due to the lack of high-quality data. The present study overcomes two challenges that many extant studies faced in evaluating the distance effect on FP use. The first challenge is the inaccuracy of the distance measurement. Although recent technological advancements have allowed many publicly available data to contain the geographical information of households, GPS coordinates are often perturbed to protect the confidentiality of respondents. Examples of such data include the Demographic and Health Survey (DHS) and the Living Standards Measurement Study (LSMS). The resulting measurement error will cause attenuation bias to the estimation of the distance effect. Many studies use DHS or LSMS data to evaluate the distance effect on FP use (Oliver, 1995; Feyisetan & Ainsworth, 1996; Thomas & Maluccio, 1996; Paul, 1991; Heard et al., 2004; Tegegne et al., 2018; Skiles et al., 2015). However, the distance effect contains biases in these studies.

The second challenge is the lack of detailed information on each health facility. The quality of a health facility can significantly influence health service utilization (Gage et al., 2018). However, obtaining information on the quality of a health facility has been difficult. For example, the census list of a health facility can provide information on the location of all health facilities, but the information contained in the list is extremely limited in evaluating the quality of each health facility. Some publicly available health facility data, such as the Service Provision Assessment (ICF, 2017), contain the detailed information of each health facility. However, these data mostly do not contain information on all health facilities.

There are only a limited number of studies that overcome these challenges to evaluate the distance effects on FP use. One such example is the study by Shiferaw et al. (2017). Using the accurate household location and detailed information on the health facility, they found that women who live close to a health facility that offers a wider range of contraceptive methods were significantly more likely to use modern contraceptives.

This study contributes to the growing literature on the effect of distance to a health facility on FP use. We overcome the above-mentioned challenges by using the unique data we collected, and evaluate the effect of distance to a certain type of health facility on contraceptive use among urban Turkish women.

2 Methods

We use two datasets for the analysis, namely, the household survey data, which contain the accurate location of households (GPS) and women's utilization of FP, and the health facility survey, which includes all facilities that women in the household survey utilized for FP services. This survey also contains the accurate location of each facility and whether each facility offers FP services.

Data are collected as part of the Willows Impact Evaluation Project, the purpose of which is to evaluate the effect of a community-based intervention on FP uptake in four countries: Ghana, Tanzania, Pakistan, and Turkey. The data we analyze in this paper are from the Istanbul area of Turkey.

This study utilizes the household survey conducted in two sites (Bağcılar and Küçükçekmece) within Istanbul between August and October 2018. Within these two sites, the sampling frame follows a three-stage random sampling design. The first stage involves randomly selecting streets, and the second stage randomly samples households on large streets. If there is more than one eligible woman, married and aged between 16 and 44, in a household, the third stage randomly selects one woman. We have collected the baseline data from the total of 4,224 married women aged between 16 and 44 from the two sites in Istanbul. The data contain detailed information on women's reproductive health around the utilization of FP and sociodemographic characteristics, as well as the accurate location (GPS coordinates) of each respondent's household.

Under the Willows Impact Evaluation Project, we also conducted the health facility survey among 35 health facilities that women in the household survey utilized for FP services. In this survey, we collected various information on the service availability and quality of each health facility. We also measured the accurate GPS coordinates of each facility. The distance from the respondents' location to each health facility is calculated, using the accurate GPS coordinates of both locations of the respondents and of the health facilities. Figure 8.1 presents the geographical distribution of women's locations and health facilities.

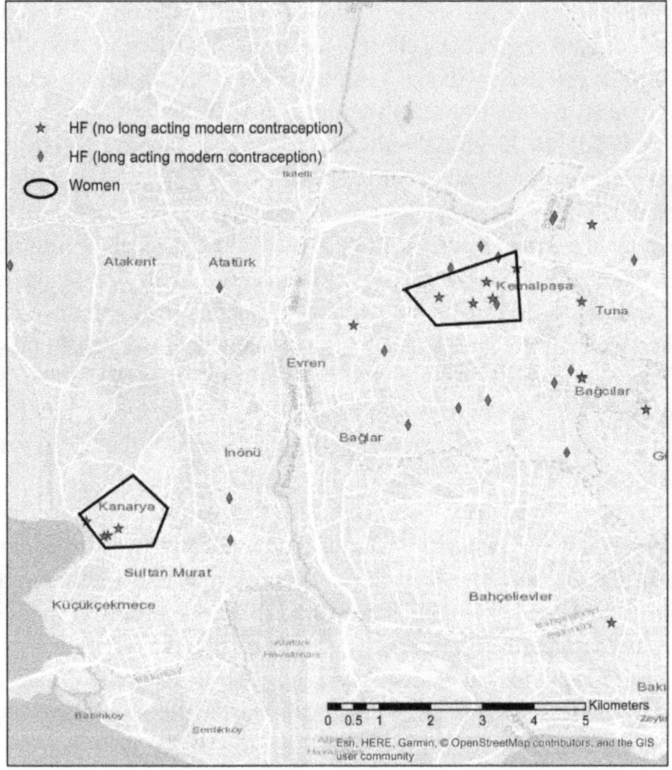

Fig. 8.1: Geographical distribution of women's locations and health facilities

2.1 Main Outcome Variables

The main outcome variable is current use of contraceptive method at the time of the interview. We differentiate contraceptive use by its type: any modern FP, short-acting modern FP, and long-acting modern FP.

2.2 Explanatory Variable

The main explanatory variable is distance to a health facility, according to its type. We categorize the health facility (HF) into two: HF where the service provision of long-acting FP is not available and HF where the service provision of long-acting FP is available. If an HF provides at least one of the long-acting FP services, namely, female sterilization, male sterilization, IUD, and implants, then it is considered an HF with long-acting FP. If none of the long-acting FP services is provided in an HF, then it is considered an HF with no long-acting FP.

Other quality measure of the health facility can influence the uptake of family planning, such as fee for the service. Among health facilities that offer long-acting FP, over 40 % of them charge for the services. In the sample, about 60 % of women go to health facilities that offer the long-acting FP services with fee, while the remaining 40 % go to health facilities without fee. Because the existence of fee does not prevent women from utilizing health facilities, we focus only on the distance aspect in this analysis to avoid unnecessarily complicating the analysis.

2.3 Statistical Analysis

To evaluate the distance effect on the utilization of FP, we first use the logistic regression in the following regression framework:

$$y_{ij} = \alpha + \beta_1 (Distance to nearest\ HF = far)_{ij} + X'\mu + \varepsilon_{ij}, \tag{1}$$

where y_{ij} is an outcome of a respondent i in a study site j, the current FP use according to its type; $(Distance to nearest\ HF = far)$ indicates if distance to the nearest HF, regardless of the availability of FP, is far from a respondent i's household. In X, we control for sociodemographic characteristics of women and household such as age, working status, education level, number of births, months since the last births, wealth level, and the site where she resides.

Next, to evaluate the differential effect of distance to an HF on FP uptake, according to the type of HF in terms of FP service availability, we use the logistic regression in the following framework:

$$\begin{aligned} y_{ij} = \alpha &+ \beta_1 (Distance\ to\ HF\ with\ no\ long-acting\ FP = far)_{ij} \\ &+ \beta_2 (Distance to HF with long-acting\ FP = far)_{ij} + X'\mu + \varepsilon_{ij}, \end{aligned} \tag{2}$$

where $(Distance to HF with no long-acting\ FP = far)$ indicates if distance to a nearest HF that does not provide long-acting FP is far from a respondent i's location. $(Distance to HF with long-acting\ FP = far)$ indicates if distance to a nearest HF that provides long-acting FP is far from a respondent i's location.

We use two cutoffs to define whether distance to an HF is far: 0.5 km and 1.5 km; we define that distance to the nearest HF is far if the distance is 500 m or more. Similarly, we define that distance to a nearest HF with no long-acting FP is far if the distance is 500 m or more. We further define that distance to such HF with long-acting FP as very far if it is 1.5 km or more. We do not have the cutoff of 1.5 km for the nearest HF and HF that does not provide long-acting FP, because the maximum distance to these HFs is less than 1.5 km (Tab. 8.1). In *X*, we control for the same sociodemographic characteristics as in the specification (1).

Tab. 8.1: Summary Statistics

Variable	**N**	**%**	**Mean**	**Std. Dev.**
Age				
16–24	449	11.36		
25–29	774	19.58		
30–34	876	22.16		
35–39	903	22.84		
40–44	951	24.06		
Working status				
Working	214	5.41		
Not working	3,739	94.59		
Education				
No education	822	20.79		
Primary	1,844	46.65		
Secondary	669	16.92		
Higher	618	15.63		
Births				
Total # births			2.32	1.52
Months since the last birth (=0 if never)			56.37	63.89
Wealth index				
Poorest	466	11.79		
Poorer	487	12.32		
Medium	954	24.13		
Richer	1,462	36.98		
Richest	584	14.77		
	Mean	Std. Dev	Min	Max
Distance (km) to				
Nearest HF	0.334	0.210	0.008	0.942
HF without long acting FP	0.355	0.207	0.008	0.942
HF with long acting FP	0.945	0.601	0.014	2.192

Notes: The sample is 3,953 women.

3 Results

Out of 4,224 women interviewed for the household survey, we use the analysis sample of 3,953 women who have complete information on the main variables. We use all 35 HFs from the health facility survey for the analysis.

Figure 8.2 presents the prevalence of contraceptive use among the sampled women. The prevalence of overall FP use was 71.9 %, of which the prevalence of long-acting modern FP use was 21.7 %, that of short-acting modern FP was 17.0 %, and that of non-modern FP was 33.2 %. Among the long-acting modern methods, the use of IUD was the most common (14.9 %), followed by female sterilization (6.9 %). Among short-acting modern methods, the use of male condom was the most common (12.4 %), followed by oral pills (4.1 %). Among non-modern FP methods, the use of withdrawal was the most common (32.5 %).

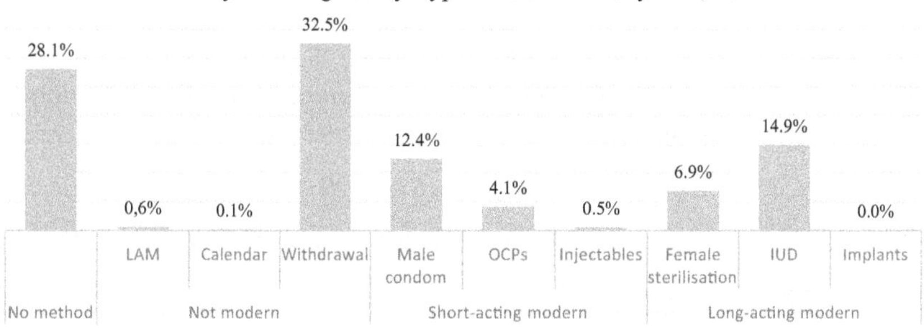

Fig. 8.2: Prevalence of FP use among women in Istanbul area, Turkey
Notes: The sample is 3,953 married women aged 16–44 in two areas in Istanbul, Turkey.

Appendix 8.1 presents the availability of FP services at HFs. Out of the total of 35 HFs in the health facility survey, 17 HFs offered the female sterilization service, 15 offered the IUD service, 12 offered the male sterilization service, and 6 HFs offered the implant service. Out of 35 HFs, condoms were available in 10 HFs, pills in 8 HFs, and injectables in 9 HFs.

Table 8.1 presents the descriptive statistics of women. The sample consisted of the higher proportion of women at older age than at younger age; 24.1 % were between 40 and 44 years old while 11.4 % were between 16 and 24 years old. Only approximately 5 % were working (5.4 %). More than one-fifths (20.8 %) had no educational attainment, and 46.7 % completed primary education. The average number of births was 2.3, and the average months since the last birth was 56 months. On average, the women in our sample were concentrated in the middle to the richer households; 24.1 % and 37.0 % were in medium and richer households, respectively. On the other hand, the proportion of women in the poorest and poorer households were 11.8 % and 12.3 %, respectively. We constructed the wealth index to be comparable with the nationally representative sample used in Turkey's DHS in 2013 (Hacettepe University Institute of Population Studies, 2014). The average distance to the nearest HF was 334 m. The distance to an HF that did not provide long-acting FP was 355 m, and the distance to an HF that provided long-acting FP was 945 m. Appendix 8.2 presents the kernel density of distance to an HF, according to the availability of FP. About half of women walk to the health facility, while a quarter of them use either public transport such as bus or private transport such as taxi, respectively.

Table 8.2 presents the main results. First, distance to an HF, regardless of its type in terms of FP availability, was not associated with the likelihood of the utilization of any modern FP (Tab. 8.2, column 1). Second, distance to an HF that did not provide long-acting FP was not associated with the uptake of short-acting FP nor long-acting FP (columns 2 and 3). On the other hand, if distance to an HF that provided long-acting FP was very far, then the odds of short-acting FP uptake was 60.1 % higher (column 2) while the odds of long-acting FP uptake is 32.9 % lower (column 3). Figure 8.3 presents the logistic regression results from Tab. 8.2 in the figure.

Tab. 8.2: Effect of distance to a health facility on modern FP use among women in Istanbul area, Turkey

	Any	**Short-acting**	**Long-acting**
	(1)	**(2)**	**(3)**
HF with not long-acting FP = Far (≥0.5km)	1.053	1.006	1.068
	[0.865,1.284]	[0.790,1.282]	[0.838,1.362]
HF with long-acting FP = Far (≥0.5km & <1.5km)	1.246	1.453***	0.998
	[0.999,1.554]	[1.101,1.918]	[0.771,1.292]
HF with long-acting FP = Very Far (≥1.5km)	1.055	1.601**	0.671**
	[0.778,1.429]	[1.100,2.328]	[0.465,0.969]
N	3953	3953	3953
covariates	X	X	X

Notes: The sample is 3,953 women. Results are based on the logistic regression of distance dummy variable on the FP use. The comparisongroup for each independent variable is the distance for each HF <0.5km. "Non long-acting HF = Far (≥1.5km)"are dropped because there is no observation with >1.5km. "Non long-acting HF=Far" takes 1 if the distance to HF with non long acting is 0.5km or more, "Long-acting HF=Far" takes 1 if the distance to HF with long-acting is (≥0.5km & <1.5km). "Long-acting HF=Very Far" takes 1 if the distance to HF with long-acting is more than 1.5km. We include the covariates in the logistic regression: age, working status, education, number of births, months since the last births (= 0 if never), wealth index, site (control/intervention). ** significant at 5 % *** significant at 1 %

Table 8.3 presents the effect of distance to an HF on the uptake of each type of FP. We found that if distance to an HF that provided long-acting FP was very far, the odds of pill uptake, one of the short-acting FP, increased by almost 2.5 folds (Tab. 8.3, column 2) while the odds of IUD uptake, one of the long-acting FP, is lower by approximately 37 % (Tab. 8.3, column 5). Figure 8.4 presents the logistic regression results from Tab. 8.3 in the figure, focusing on pills and IUD.

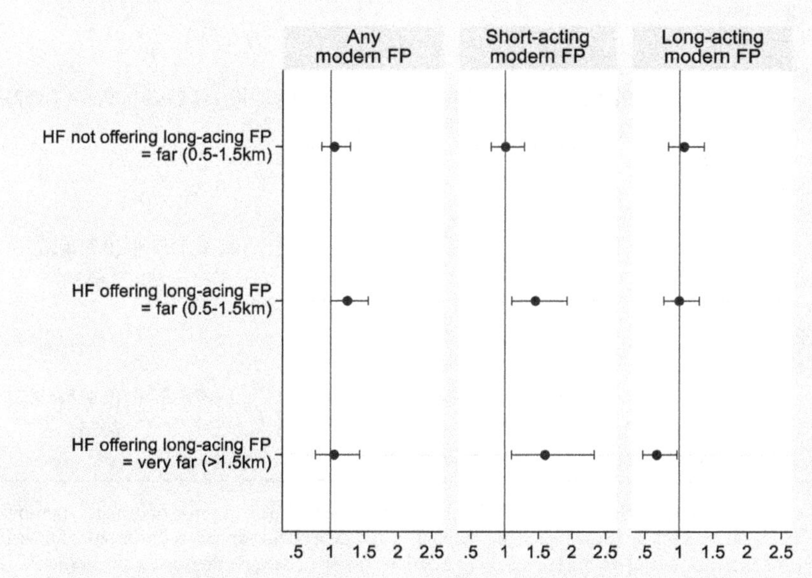

Fig. 8.3: Effect of distance to a health facility on FP use among women in Istanbul area, Turkey

Notes: The sample is 3,953 women. The coefficients are based on the logistic regression of distance dummy variable on the FP use. The comparison group for each independent variable is the distance for each HF <0.5km. "Non long-acting HF = Very Far (1.5km)" is dropped because there is no observation with >1.5km. "Non long-acting HF=Far" takes 1 if the distance to HF with non long acting is 0.5km or more, "Long-acting HF=Far" takes 1 if the distance to HF with long-acting is (≥0.5km & <1.5km). "Long-acting HF=Very Far" takes 1 if the distance to HF with long-acting is more than 1.5km. We include the covariates in the logistic regression: age, working status, education, number of births, months since the last births (=0 if never), wealth index, site (control/ intervention).

Tab. 8.3: Effect of distance to a health facility on modern FP use among women in Istanbul area, Turkey

	Non-modern	Short-acting modern		Long-acting modern	
	Withdrawal	**Pills**	**Condoms**	**Female sterlization**	**IUD**
	(1)	**(2)**	**(3)**	**(4)**	**(5)**
HF with not long-acting FP = Far (≥0.5km)	1.083	0.856	1.017	0.667	1.272
	[0.891,1.317]	[0.549,1.334]	[0.771,1.340]	[0.434,1.024]	[0.974,1.662]
HF with long-acting FP = Far (≥0.5km & <1.5km)	0.972	2.276***	1.094	1.111	0.949
	[0.770,1.227]	[1.359,3.813]	[0.791,1.512]	[0.735,1.679]	[0.710,1.270]
HF with long-acting FP = Very Far (≥1.5km)	1.153	2.467***	1.170	0.858	0.633**
	[0.846,1.573]	[1.247,4.883]	[0.759,1.806]	[0.467,1.579]	[0.418,0.957]
N	3953	3953	3953	3953	3953
covariates	X	X	X	X	X

Notes: The sample is 3,953 women. Results are based on the logistic regression of distance dummy variable on the FP use. The comparisongroup for each independent variable is the distance for each HF <0.5km. "Non long-acting HF = Far (≥1.5km)"are dropped because there is no observation with >1.5km. "Non long-acting HF=Far" takes 1 if the distance to HF with non long acting is 0.5km or more, "Long-acting HF=Far" takes 1 if the distance to HF with long-acting is (≥0.5km & <1.5km). "Long-acting HF=Very Far" takes 1 if the distance to HF with long-acting is more than 1.5km. We include the covariates in the logistic regression: age, working status, education, number of births, months since the last births (=0 if never), wealth index, site (control/intervention). ** significant at 5 % *** significant at 1 %

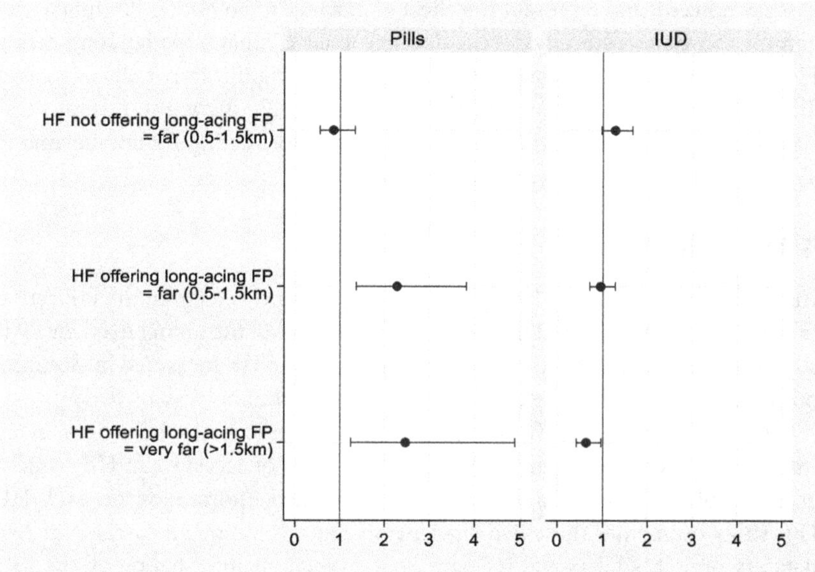

Fig. 8.4: Effect of distance to a health facility on FP use (specific) among women in Istanbul area, Turkey

Notes: The sample is 3,953 women. The coefficients are based on the logistic regression of distance dummy variable on the FP use. The comparison group for each independent variable is the distance for each HF <0.5km. "Non long-acting HF = Very Far (1.5km)" is dropped because there is no observation with >1.5km. "Non long-acting HF=Far" takes 1 if the distance to HF with non long acting is 0.5km or more, "Long-acting HF=Far" takes 1 if the distance to HF with long-acting is (≥0.5km & <1.5km). "Long-acting HF=Very Far" takes 1 if the distance to HF with long-acting is more than 1.5km. We include the covariates in the logistic regression: age, working status, education, number of births, months since the last births (=0 if never), wealth index, site (control/ intervention).

Appendices 8.3 and 8.4 present the effect of distance to an HF on FP uptake, based on the wealth level of the women's households. The effect of very-far distance to an HF that provided long-acting FP on the uptake of long-acting FP was negative and statistically significant among the poor (Appendix 8.4, column 6), while the relationship was not statistically significant among the non-poor (column 3). On the other hand, the effect of very-far distance to an HF that provided long-acting FP on the uptake of short-acting FP was insignificant among both the poor and the non-poor.

Appendices 5 and 6 present the effect of distance to an HF on FP uptake, according to women's ethnicity. If the distance to an HF that provided long-acting FP is very far, the odds of long-acting FP uptake are significantly reduced among Turkish women, but not among Kurdish women. Similarly, the distance was significantly associated with the higher odds of short-acting FP uptake among Turkish women, but not among Kurdish women.

4 Discussion

Although the past decades have observed a rapid improvement in the utilization of contraceptive use around the world, the prevalence of the unmet need for FP is still high. This paper evaluates the effect of access to an HF, measured by distance, on contraceptive use among married women in the Istanbul area of Turkey.

Although access to an HF is a well-studied barrier to health behaviors, many existing studies face challenges in the measurement of access to an HF, namely, accuracy of distance to an HF and lack of detailed information on each HF. Our study overcomes these two challenges using two unique datasets. Our two datasets, household data and HF data, contain accurate information on the GPS coordinates of each respondent's location and of each HF. Our health facility survey also contains detailed information about the availability of FP service.

Among our sample women, the prevalence of overall FP use is 71.9 %. The most common contraceptive method is withdrawal (32.5 %), followed by IUD (14.9 %), one of the long-acting modern methods, and male condom (12.4 %), one of the short-acting modern methods.

We find that the effect of distance to an HF on contraceptive use differs, according to the type of HF and the type of FP methods the respondents use. First, distance to an HF that does not provide long-acting FP is not associated with the likelihood that the respondents use contraceptives of any type. It is not associated with the uptake of long-acting FP such as IUD because such HFs that do not provide long-acting FP cannot provide services necessary for women to have long-acting FP, such as the insertion of IUD, which is the most common long-acting method in the area.

Similarly, distance to an HF that does not provide long-acting FP is also not associated with the utilization of short-acting FP such as condom. This is presumably because in Istanbul, many FP commodities that are short-acting methods are available outside of HFs, without women needing to obtain a prescription for the purchase of these methods. For example, condoms are available in shops and pharmacies. Other short-acting FP methods such as oral pills are also purchasable at pharmacies without prescription.

Second, longer distance to an HF that provides long-acting FP is negatively associated with long-acting contraceptive use. Our result indicates that access to an HF and availability of services at the HF are both important predictors of the utilization of FP. This result is consistent with some of the existing studies. For example, Shiferaw et al. (2017) found that women who live close to facilities that offer a wider range of contraceptive methods were significantly more likely to use modern contraceptives.

Longer distance to an HF that offers long-acting FP is, on the contrary, positively associated with the uptake of short-acting FP methods. This result implies that the respondents substitute long-acting FP methods with short-acting FP ones when access to an HF that offers long-acting FP is difficult. As we described above in the Results section, the utilization of short-acting methods such as condoms and pills is not dependent on the service availability at HFs.

Overall, we observe substitution behaviors in terms of choice of contraceptive methods, from long-acting to short-acting, among Turkish women in urban Istanbul, when they are faced with the difficult accessibility to HFs that offer long-acting methods.

Although urban Turkish women mitigate the risk of unintended pregnancy by shifting from long-acting to short-acting methods when access to a long-acting method is difficult, this barrier to long-acting methods still exposes women to the risk of unintended pregnancy because short-acting methods have higher discontinuation rate (Hubacher et al., 2017). Furthermore, among the vulnerable population such as the poor, longer distance to an HF that provides long-acting FP only decreases the uptake of long-acting methods without increasing the uptake of short-acting ones. This result indicates that the poor have the higher risk of unintended pregnancy due to longer distance to an adequate HF.

5 Conclusions

This paper evaluates the effect of distance to HFs, according to their types based on FP service availability, on contraceptive use among married women in Istanbul. We find that longer distance to an HF that provides long-acting FP is negatively associated with the likelihood that women use long-acting FP. On the other hand, it is positively associated with the likelihood that women use short-acting FP. Distance to an HF is an important and significant barrier to contraceptive use if the facility offers the services that women desire. If access to an HF that provides long-acting FP is difficult, women substitute the utilization of a long-acting FP method with a short-acting one, which is available outside of HFs without prescription, but with less efficacy to prevent unwanted pregnancy. Our results imply that the policy should prioritize to enhance the access to the long-acting FP among the poor.

References

Ali, M., Farron, M., Dilip, T. R., & Folz, R. (2018). Assessment of family planning service availability and readiness in 10 African countries. *Global Health: Science and Practice, 6*(3), 473–483.

Cahill, N., Sonneveldt, E., Stover, J., Weinberger, M., Williamson, J., Wei, C., Brown, W., & Alkema, L. (2018). Modern contraceptive use, unmet need, and demand satisfied among women of reproductive age who are married or in a union in the focus countries of the Family Planning 2020 initiative: A systematic analysis using the Family Planning Estimation Tool. *The Lancet, 391*(10123), 870–882.

Feyisetan, B. J., & Ainsworth, M. (1996). Contraceptive use and the quality, price, and availability of family planning in Nigeria. *The World Bank Economic Review, 10*(1), 159- 187.

Gage, A. D., Leslie, H. H., Bitton, A., Jerome, J. G., Joseph, J. P., Thermidor, R., & Kruk, M. E. (2018). Does quality influence utilization of primary health care? Evidence from Haiti. *Globalization and Health, 14*(1), 59.

Hacettepe University Institute of Population Studies. (2014). *2013 Turkey Demographic and Health Survey. Hacettepe University Institute of Population Studies*, T.R. Ministry of Development and TÜBITAK.

Heard, N. J., Larsen, U., & Hozumi, D. (2004). Investigating access to reproductive health services using GIS: Proximity to services and the use of modern contraceptives in Malawi. *African Journal of Reproductive Health, 8*(2), 164–179.

Hubacher, D., Spector, H., Monteith, C., Chen, P. L., & Hart, C. (2017). Long-acting reversible contraceptive acceptability and unintended pregnancy among women presenting for short-acting methods: A randomized patient preference trial. *American Journal of Obstetrics and Gynecology, 216*(2), 101–109.

ICF. (2017). *The DHS Program: SPA Overview.* https://dhsprogram.com/methodology/Survey-Types/SPA.cfm

Karra, M., Fink, G., & Canning, D. (2017). Facility distance and child mortality: A multi-country study of health facility access, service utilization, and child health outcomes. *International Journal of Epidemiology, 46*(3), 817–826.

Oliver, R. (1995). *Contraceptive use in Ghana: The role of service availability, quality, and price*. The World Bank. https://doi.org/10.1596/0-8213-3020-9

Paul, B. K. (1991). Family planning availability and contraceptive use in rural Bangladesh: An examination of the distance decay effect. *Socio-Economic Planning Sciences, 25*(4), 269- 282.

Shiferaw, S., Spigt, M., Seme, A., Amogne, A., Skrøvseth, S., Desta, S., Radloff, S., Tsui, A., & GeertJan, D. (2017). Does proximity of women to facilities with better choice o f contraceptives affect their contraceptive utilization in rural Ethiopia?. *PLOS ONE, 12*(11), e0187311.

Skiles, M. P., Cunningham, M., Inglis, A., Wilkes, B., Hatch, B., Bock, A., & Barden-O'Fallon, J. (2015). The effect of access to contraceptive services on injectable use and demand for family planning in Malawi. *International Perspectives on Sexual and Reproductive Health, 41*(1), 20–30.

Tegegne, T. K., Chojenta, C., Loxton, D., Smith, R., & Kibret, K. T. (2018). The impact of geographic access on institutional delivery care use in low and middle-income countries: Systematic review and meta-analysis. *PLOS ONE, 13*(8), e0203130.

Thomas, D., & Maluccio, J. (1996). Fertility, contraceptive choice, and public policy in Zimbabwe. *The World Bank Economic Review, 10*(1), 189–222.

Yao, J., Murray, A. T., Agadjanian, V., & Hayford, S. R. (2012). Geographic influences on sexual and reproductive health service utilization in rural Mozambique. *Applied Geography, 32*(2), 601–607.

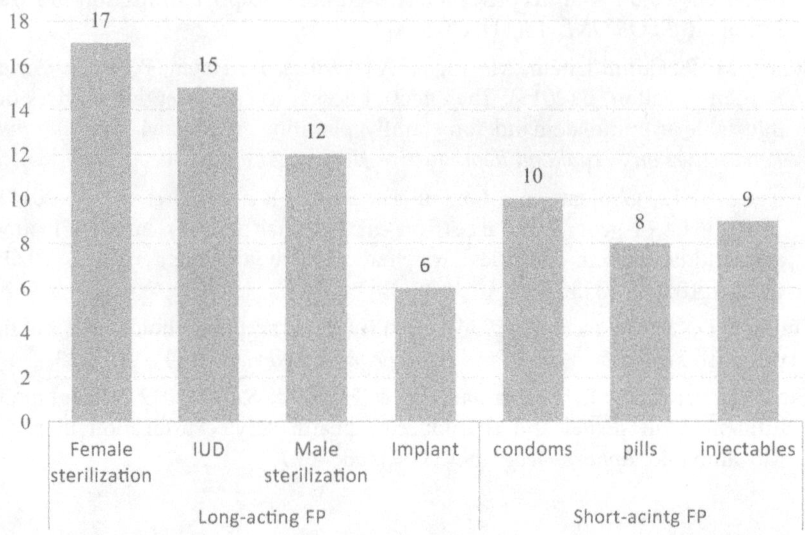

Appendix 8.1: Breakdown of health facilities by type of FP provision, used by women in Istanbul area, Turkey

Notes: The total number of health facilities is 35. The number in the figure indicates the number of health facilities which provide each of FP methods.

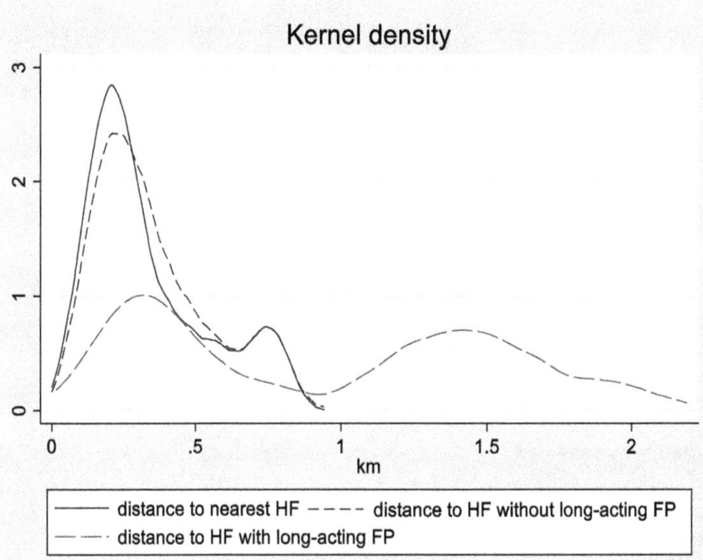

Appendix 8.2: Distribution of distance to a health facility used by women in Istanbul area, Turkey

Notes: The sample is 3,953 women.

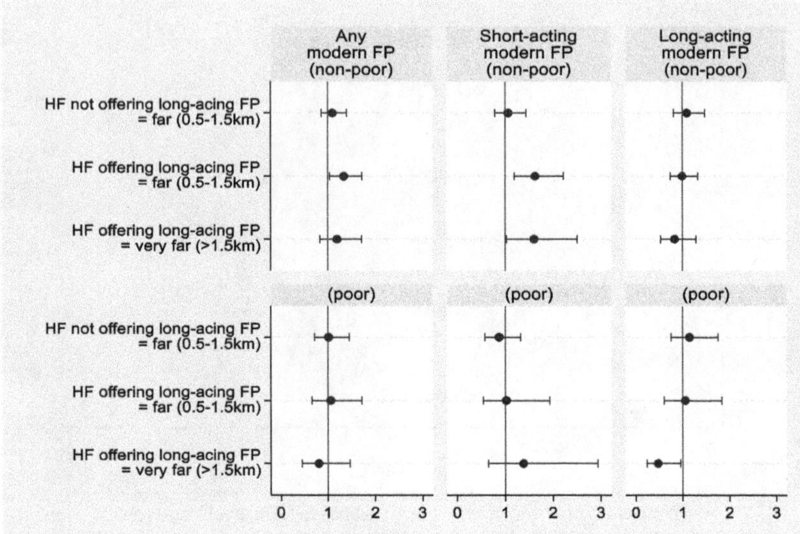

Appendix 8.3: Effect of distance to a health facility on FP use by wealth status

Notes: The sample is 3,953 women. A women belongs to "Poor" if the wealth index for her household is poorest or poorer. The coefficients are based on the logistic regression of distance dummy variable on the FP use. The comparison group for each independent variable is the distance for each HF <0.5km. "Non long-acting HF = Very Far (1.5km)" is dropped because there is no observation with >1.5km. "Non long-acting HF=Far" takes 1 if the distance to HF with non long acting is 0.5km or more, "Long-acting HF=Far" takes 1 if the distance to HF with long-acting is (≥0.5km & <1.5km). "Long-acting HF=Very Far" takes 1 if the distance to HF with long-acting is more than 1.5km. We include the covariates in the logistic regression: age, working status, education, number of births, months since the last births (=0 if never), site (control/intervention).

Appendix 8.4: Effect of distance to a health facility on modern FP use by wealth status (specific, Full model)

	Any	Short-acting	Long-acting	Any	Short-acting	Long-acting
	Non-Poor			**Poor (poorest / poorer)**		
	(1)	(2)	(3)	(4)	(5)	(6)
HF with not long-acting FP = Far (≥0.5km)	1.097	1.063	1.094	1.015	0.871	1.147
	[0.862,1.396]	[0.786,1.438]	[0.810,1.476]	[0.712,1.446]	[0.575,1.321]	[0.748,1.758]
HF with long-acting FP = Far (≥0.5km & <1.5km)	1.336**	1.626***	0.992	1.059	1.022	1.054
	[1.039,1.716]	[1.193,2.217]	[0.740,1.331]	[0.655,1.713]	[0.542,1.927]	[0.605,1.835]
HF with long-acting FP = Very Far (≥1.5km)	1.194	1.602**	0.828	0.802	1.375	0.470**
	[0.832,1.712]	[1.025,2.505]	[0.533,1.286]	[0.441,1.460]	[0.645,2.933]	[0.231,0.954]
N	3000	3000	3000	953	953	953
covariates	X	X	X	X	X	X

Notes: The sample is 3,953 women. Results are based on the logistic regression of distance dummy variable on the FP use. The comparisongroup for each independent variable is the distance for each HF <0.5km. "Non long-acting HF = Far (≥1.5km)"are dropped because there is no observation with >1.5km. "Non long-acting HF=Far" takes 1 if the distance to HF with non long acting is 0.5km or more, "Long-acting HF=Far" takes 1 if the distance to HF with long-acting is (≥0.5km & <1.5km). "Long-acting HF=Very Far" takes 1 if the distance to HF with long-acting is more than 1.5km. We include the covariates in the logistic regression: age, working status, education, number of births, months since the last births (=0 if never), wealth index, site (control/ intervention). ** significant at 5 % *** significant at 1 %

JULIA KATHERINE ROHR

9 Contraceptive Choices and Fertility Preferences

Abstract: This chapter provides an overview of available contraceptive methods, contraceptive decision-making, and fertility preferences in poorer working-class areas of Istanbul (Bağcılar and Küçükçekmece). First, we give a brief overview of the knowledge of different types of contraception, sources of information, and frequency of use. Next, we look in-depth to understand the reasons that drive choice of specific contraceptive methods, and what predicts the use of permanent, long-acting reversible, short acting, and traditional methods. The determinants of method choice that we will examine include fertility preferences, access to healthcare, receipt of counseling, availability of preferred methods, and husband's preferences.

Keywords : Choice of contraceptives, long-acting contraceptives, fertility preference, male sterilization, female sterilization, injectables, boy preference.

1 Introduction

Worldwide, women are more frequently choosing contraception to limit or space births. Contraceptives are used by the majority of married women in almost all regions of the world, although the types of methods used and prevalence of use vary widely across regions and countries. The unmet need for family planning still persists globally, with at least one in ten married women in most regions of the world continuing to have unmet need (UN, 2015). Ideally, the choice of a contraceptive method should be influenced by a woman's assessment of her needs compared to all available options. Choosing a contraceptive method that is well suited to meet a woman's preferences can lead to more accurate and continuous use of the method (Marshall et al., 2015). However, even in contexts where modern contraception is freely available, misinformation, lack of awareness, and fear of judgment or embarrassment can interfere with women's uptake of contraceptive methods (Foster & Doci, 2017).

In Turkey, there is high awareness of contraception and met need for contraception overall, with unmet need found among 6 % of married women, as reported in the Turkey Demographic and Health Survey. The majority of married women (76.7 %) report having ever used a modern contraceptive method, while 47.4 % currently use a modern method. In Turkey, the desire for fertility is correlated largely with younger age and a lower number of children. Despite a low overall proportion of women with unmet need across the country, the need for improvement in the uptake and use of effective contraceptive methods remains. The total desired fertility rate in Turkey of 1.9 is lower than the actual fertility rate of 2.3, and 12.5 % of most recent births have been reported as unwanted. Reports of unwanted births were even higher for women with 4 or more children, among whom 40 % said their most recent birth was unwanted (DHS, 2014).

The trends in the use of contraception and unmet need in Turkey also show important disparities according to socioeconomic status. Higher use of modern contraception is correlated with more education and wealth, and the highest amount of unmet need for family planning is found among the youngest, least educated, and least wealthy women (DHS, 2014). Recent research from Turkey demonstrates that accurate use of family planning services increases with improvements in women's education, wealth, and employment (Çalıkoğlu et al., 2018; Özdemir et al., 2019). Attitudes toward family planning also improve with education for both the woman and her husband (Ayaz & Efe, 2009).

When considering barriers to contraception use in Turkey, lack of knowledge or appropriate counseling, issues regarding access and convenience, and husbands' attitudes may all play a role. Most modern contraceptive methods in Turkey are accessed through the public sector (55.9 %), while 37 % are accessed through the private sector and 6.6 % through shops, mainly for purchasing condoms. Among those who access contraceptive methods through the private sector, 23.2 % go to pharmacies for pills or condoms (DHS, 2014), yet half of the pharmacists in the Istanbul region have never received training specific to contraception (Özaydın et al., 2020). Providing pharmacists with in-service training on contraceptive counseling has been identified as a potential area for improvement to reach women with contraceptive counseling services (Özaydin et al., 2020). Lack of awareness of methods has also been identified among men in Turkey as an obstacle to contraception use (Yılmazel et al., 2019). Women report having difficulty accessing family planning services at health centers due to gender-related barriers as well as poor provision of contraceptives and consultations (Yücel et al., 2020). Among women using contraception, ease of availability is a commonly stated reason for method choice (25 %) (Çalıkoğlu et al., 2018). Male partners are reported as a significant barrier to contraception only in some cases. Among non-users of contraception, husbands' opposition has been reported as the most important reason for nonuse among 7 % of young married women aged 15–29 years (DHS, 2014). Most male partners report involvement in family planning services with their spouse (75.5 %), and the majority of men report that they approve of contraceptive use, although many say women are mostly expected to shoulder the responsibility for using contraception. The main obstacles to contraception reported by men included having no knowledge, being sinful, disadvantages of the methods, and lack of accessibility (Yılmazel et al., 2019). Male support for contraception varies by age, education and occupation and has an impact on spouses' attitudes toward family planning (Yılmazel et al., 2019; Ayaz & Efe, 2009).

Current research from Turkey makes it clear that some women who need family planning do not use it and that there are disparities across the population, putting vulnerable women, especially those who are younger, less wealthy and less educated, at higher risk. In this chapter, we explore contraceptive choices among women living in economically disadvantaged neighborhoods of Istanbul. This population, which tends to be poor but geographically close to major hospitals and healthcare services, is interesting to study for gaining insight into which methods vulnerable women choose and are able to access. We have the following specific objectives: (1) describe the awareness and use of different types of contraceptive methods among this population and (2) examine factors that impact contraceptive use overall as well as the choice of specific methods, including (a) women's concerns and obstacles regarding contraception use, (b) women's fertility desires, and (c) their husbands' desires and support.

2 Study Population

The study took place in two districts in Istanbul that are west of the city center, including Fatih and Demirkapı mahalles in Bağcılar and Kanarya mahalle in Küçükçekmece. Both sites tend to be low income, with a large Kurdish population, and receive migrants mainly from Eastern and Southeastern Anatolia. A cross-sectional survey took place in these neighborhoods from March – June 2018. The survey was conducted in person in Turkish by female interviewers and included questions about basic demographic information, reproduction, pregnancy history, contraceptive use, marriage, fertility preferences, and other women's health topics. Women were eligible for the survey if they spoke Turkish, were between the ages of 17–44 years old, were married, and resided in a selected household. Using the National Statistics Institute address list, we randomly sampled streets at each site, and the interviewers approached the households to determine whether a woman eligible for interview resided in the household and was available. For large streets, a subsample of household addresses was randomly selected prior to the fieldwork. Some households refused to speak to the interviewers, had invalid addresses, or were not available. Among the resulting 8,100 women asked to participate in the survey, 50.9 % completed the survey, 40.4 % were not available after three attempts, and 7.5 % refused to participate.

The final study sample consisted of 4,224 women, half living in Bağcılar and half in Küçükçekmece.

3 Analytic Methods

3.1 Univariate Analyses

We give a brief overview of the frequency of the responses to questions about awareness of different types of contraception, sources of information, and use of different methods. Statistical analyses include tabulations and comparisons between groups using chi-square tests. Univariate analyses are also used to examine the frequencies of the features of contraception women considered most important and the reported obstacles in obtaining contraception, as well as the desire for children and prevalence of unmet need. Husband support is also examined with cross tabulations and chi-square tests to explore associations between husband support and other characteristics, including age at first cohabitation, age difference between the woman and her husband, kin marriage, woman's age, and husband's desire for children relative to the woman's desire (whether he wants more, fewer, or the same number of children as the woman wants, or she does not know).

3.2 Multivariate Models

In multivariate models, we explore predictors of (1) the current use of any contraception and of any modern contraception, (2) desire for more children, and (3) unmet need for contraception. Regression analyses are performed using a modified Poisson model with robust error variances to estimate the relative risks with confidence intervals for each of these outcomes (Zou, 2004). Models predicting relative risks rather than odds ratios are more appropriate for these data given that many of the outcomes are not rare. Demographic characteristics are considered in all models. Predictors of current contraception use and modern contraception use include demographic characteristics, including education and wealth, as well as awareness of types, sources of method, sources of knowledge, and reception of counseling during recent visits to the health facility to investigate how the knowledge and reception of information regarding contraception may influence the use of modern methods. Predictors considered in the model for the unmet need for family planning also include the husband's support for the woman's contraceptive choices and the husband's desire for children relative to the woman to provide further insight into how husbands' attitudes may impact meeting women's need for contraception.

3.3 Models for the Choice of a Specific Contraceptive Method

Finally, we examine trends in the choices of specific types of contraceptive methods using two methods. First, using modified Poisson regression models as described above, we predict the relative use of each major contraceptive type as the outcome: female sterilization, inter-uterine devices (IUDs), injectables, pills, condoms, withdrawal, other traditional methods, and no methods. Second, we calculate the age-standardized prevalence of each of these contraceptive types stratified by different characteristics using direct standardization in STATA. This method allows us to calculate and visualize the prevalence of the use of specific contraceptive types for different segments of the population while accounting for age variation by standardizing the age distribution of the study population. The following variables and characteristics are considered in these models to predict the use of specific contraceptive types and as stratifying variables in the calculation of age standardized rates of use of specific contraceptive types.

1. Factors relating to knowledge and awareness: (a) number of contraceptive types the woman is aware of;
2. Factors relating to women's obstacles and concerns: (b) the most important feature of contraception women report; (c) commonly reported obstacles to obtaining family planning advice or treatment; (d) worry about the financial support of a child; (e) health insurance coverage; (f) women's report that they would not look forward to telling their parents about the next or current pregnancy; (g) women's report that they would not look forward to telling their husband about the next or current pregnancy;
3. Factors relating to fertility desire and husband support: (h) women's report that the husband does not support them in their choice of contraception; (i) fertility desire (wants to limit, wants to space, wants more children soon, or infecund); and (j) the husband's desire for children relative to the woman's desire.

Regression models predicting contraceptive type are adjusted for demographic characteristics found to be significantly associated with overall modern contraceptive use. Interaction terms are also considered for women's fertility desire and husbands' fertility desire, to see whether the impact of women's fertility desire on the use of contraception differs by husbands' desire for children, as well as interaction between women's fertility desire and husbands' support, to see whether the impact of women's fertility desire on the use of contraception differs according to husbands' support.

3.4 Definition of Variables

Throughout the analyses, modern contraception includes female sterilization, IUDs, injectables, pills, condoms, female condoms, and emergency contraception. Traditional contraception includes withdrawal, the calendar method, the lactational amenorrhea method (LAM), and other traditional methods. Models for specific contraceptive types are divided into female sterilization, IUD, injectables, pills, condoms (including female condoms, which were only reported by 2 women), withdrawal, and other traditional methods (including LAM, calendar method, and other traditional use, which were reported by <1 % of women). Only one woman reported emergency contraception and was not included in the analyses for models of specific contraceptive types.

Unmet need for family planning was calculated using the DHS algorithm (Bradley et al., 2012) to categorize women into using contraception to limit, using contraception to space, unmet need for limiting, unmet need for spacing, no unmet need (woman wants a child within 2 years), or infecund. Family planning need can be met with traditional or modern contraceptive methods. The desire to limit childbirth implies that the woman wants no more children, and the desire to space implies that the woman does not want another child within the next 2 years.

Other covariates in the models include education level and wealth index. The education category is divided to match the education categories reported in the Turkey DHS. The wealth index is calculated using principal components analysis to be comparable to the DHS national wealth quintiles.

4 Results

4.1 Awareness and Use of Methods

First, we examine how information and awareness about contraception may impact women's choices and trends in use. We also consider how socioeconomic factors, including education, work status and wealth, may impact awareness and use of contraception. In the study population of 4,224 women, 71 % of women were currently using any form of contraception, and 80 % had ever used contraception to attempt to limit or space births. The types of contraception most commonly currently used were withdrawal (32 %), IUD (15 %), condoms (12 %), female sterilization (7 %), and pills (4 %). Other types currently used included injectables, female condom, calendar method, LAM (all <1 %), and emergency contraception (currently used by one woman). The prevalence of current modern contraceptive use was 38 % and was more common among women who were older, had a primary school education, and had more previous births (Tab. 9.1). Women with lower educational attainment had significantly lower use of modern contraception in the regression models than women who had completed high school (adjusted risk ratio [aRR] for no formal education/primary incomplete compared to completed high school = 0.72, 95 % CI: 0.63–0.83), even after adjusting for other characteristics (age, wealth quintile, work status and reception of contraceptive counseling in the last 2 years). When further examining women's employment and wealth, we found that women's work status was not associated with contraceptive use in the adjusted regression models, but the wealth index had an impact. The poorest wealth quintile had a slightly higher likelihood of using modern contraception than the wealthiest group (aRR: 1.17, 95 % CI: 1.02–1.35), perhaps indicating that women who are most concerned with the financial implications of having a child are more likely to use contraception. Age, education, wealth and lifetime births were all significantly associated with contraceptive use and were adjusted for in all multivariate models predicting contraceptive use.

Tab. 9.1: Women's characteristics and current contraceptive use

	Nonuser	**Current modern user**	**Current traditional user**
	1,213	**1,617**	**1,371**
Age			
16–19	44 (3.6 %)	4 (0.2 %)	4 (0.3 %)
20–24	235 (19.4 %)	86 (5.3 %)	111 (8.1 %)
25–29	283 (23.3 %)	280 (17.3 %)	269 (19.6 %)
30–34	220 (18.1 %)	386 (23.9 %)	314 (22.9 %)
-39	180 (14.8 %)	441 (27.3 %)	332 (24.2 %)
40–44	251 (20.7 %)	420 (26.0 %)	341 (24.9 %)
Level of education			
None/Primary incomplete	247 (20.4 %)	338 (21.0 %)	280 (20.5 %)
Primary school	476 (39.3 %)	774 (48.0 %)	693 (50.7 %)
Secondary school	237 (19.6 %)	267 (16.6 %)	221 (16.2 %)
High school and higher	250 (20.7 %)	234 (14.5 %)	173 (12.7 %)
Place of birth			
Istanbul	469 (38.8 %)	483 (30.1 %)	355 (26.0 %)
Turkey outside of Istanbul	704 (58.2 %)	1,093 (68.1 %)	988 (72.5 %)
Outside of Turkey	36 (3.0 %)	29 (1.8 %)	20 (1.5 %)
Ethnic group			
Turkish	750 (62.0 %)	942 (58.5 %)	793 (58.0 %)
Kurdish	359 (29.7 %)	542 (33.6 %)	439 (32.1 %)
Arabic	20 (1.7 %)	13 (0.8 %)	8 (0.6 %)

(Continued)

Tab. 9.1: Continued

	Nonuser	**Current modern user**	**Current traditional user**
None	79 (6.5 %)	110 (6.8 %)	126 (9.2 %)
Other	2 (0.2 %)	4 (0.2 %)	2 (0.1 %)
Current work status			
No	1,117 (92.5 %)	1,532 (95.0 %)	1,311 (95.8 %)
Yes	90 (7.5 %)	80 (5.0 %)	57 (4.2 %)
Wealth index			
Poorest	136 (11.4 %)	219 (13.7 %)	141 (10.4 %)
Poorer	138 (11.5 %)	206 (12.9 %)	168 (12.4 %)
Middle	270 (22.6 %)	368 (23.0 %)	361 (26.6 %)
Richer	460 (38.5 %)	573 (35.8 %)	500 (36.9 %)
Richest	192 (16.1 %)	235 (14.7 %)	185 (13.7 %)
Number of years in current neighborhood			
<1 year	95 (8.0 %)	43 (2.7 %)	40 (2.9 %)
1–2 years	145 (12.3 %)	54 (3.4 %)	61 (4.5 %)
2–5 years	259 (21.9 %)	228 (14.4 %)	212 (15.6 %)
5–10 years	311 (26.3 %)	475 (30.0 %)	432 (31.8 %)
>10 years	371 (31.4 %)	782 (49.4 %)	614 (45.2 %)
Age at first marriage/ cohabitation (years)			
≤19	390 (33.0 %)	754 (47.2 %)	595 (44.0 %)
20–24	559 (47.3 %)	666 (41.7 %)	594 (44.0 %)
25–29	178 (15.1 %)	155 (9.7 %)	134 (9.9 %)
30+	55 (4.7 %)	23 (1.4 %)	28 (2.1 %)
Age at first birth (years)			
≤19	171 (21.3 %)	447 (29.1 %)	350 (27.0 %)
20–24	363 (45.2 %)	778 (50.7 %)	663 (51.1 %)
25–29	190 (23.7 %)	261 (17.0 %)	241 (18.6 %)
30+	79 (9.8 %)	49 (3.2 %)	43 (3.3 %)
Lifetime births			
0	379 (31.4 %)	52 (3.2 %)	47 (3.4 %)
1	337 (27.9 %)	163 (10.1 %)	225 (16.4 %)
2	261 (21.6 %)	537 (33.4 %)	474 (34.6 %)
3	136 (11.3 %)	460 (28.6 %)	359 (26.2 %)
4	55 (4.6 %)	225 (14.0 %)	162 (11.8 %)
5+	39 (3.2 %)	172 (10.7 %)	101 (7.4 %)

* Note: Current contraceptive type missing for 23 women who are not displayed in this table.

Most women had awareness of the most commonly used contraceptive types, yet there was room for improvement in knowledge of the less commonly used types, particularly among women with lower education. Awareness of the following methods was significantly higher among those with higher education in chi-square analyses ($p < 0.05$): male sterilization, injectables, implants, pills, condoms, female condoms, spermicides, calendar/rhythm method, and emergency contraception (Tab. 9.2). Knowledge of more types of contraceptive methods was not associated with traditional method use but was associated with higher use of modern contraception after adjusting for age, education wealth, number of lifetime births, and recent reception of contraceptive counseling. For every additional contraceptive method that a woman was aware of, the relative use of modern contraception increased by 6 % (aRR: 1.06, 95 % CI: 1.04–1.08).

Tab. 9.2: Women's awareness of contraceptive methods by education level

	Education level				
Have you heard of …	**None/ Primary incomplete**	**Primary school**	**Secondary school**	**High school and higher**	**Chi-square p-value**
	867	**1,955**	**727**	**664**	
Female sterilization	827 (95.5 %)	1,871 (96.0 %)	691 (95.2 %)	643 (97.4 %)	0.15
Male sterilization	830 (96.0 %)	1,911 (98.2 %)	706 (97.2 %)	647 (98.2 %)	0.004
IUDs	837 (96.8 %)	1,913 (98.3 %)	707 (97.4 %)	648 (98.3 %)	0.054
Injectables	612 (70.7 %)	1,528 (78.5 %)	575 (79.2 %)	556 (84.4 %)	<0.001
Implants	172 (19.9 %)	453 (23.3 %)	170 (23.5 %)	213 (32.4 %)	<0.001
Pills	834 (96.3 %)	1,904 (97.8 %)	714 (98.3 %)	648 (98.5 %)	0.014
Condoms	838 (96.8 %)	1,911 (98.2 %)	712 (98.1 %)	651 (98.8 %)	0.032
Female condoms	160 (18.5 %)	329 (16.9 %)	103 (14.2 %)	151 (22.9 %)	<0.001
Spermicides	138 (16.0 %)	287 (14.8 %)	93 (12.8 %)	143 (21.7 %)	<0.001
LAM	706 (81.7 %)	1,567 (80.5 %)	574 (79.1 %)	524 (79.5 %)	0.55
Calendar method	417 (48.2 %)	1,102 (56.7 %)	466 (64.3 %)	470 (71.3 %)	<0.001
Withdrawal	840 (97.0 %)	1,901 (97.7 %)	710 (97.9 %)	647 (98.2 %)	0.43
Emergency contraception	361 (41.7 %)	1,006 (51.8 %)	396 (54.6 %)	429 (65.2 %)	<0.001

*Note: 11 women with missing data on education level not displayed.

Further examination of counseling and sources of information revealed the importance of counseling at health centers and the potential for improvement in reaching women for counseling. Overall, reports of visits to health facilities in the previous 2 years were high (81 %), and among those who had not visited a health facility in recent years, the most commonly stated reason was that they had no need for a visit. Women who had visited a health facility in the last 2 years but had not received counseling were less likely to use modern contraception than women who had received counseling or women who had not recently visited a health facility. Women who had visited but had not received counseling at a visit to a health facility in the last 2 years were more likely to use a traditional contraceptive method than women who had received counseling (aRR for traditional method use for those not counseled compared to those counseled: 1.51, 95 % CI: 1.27–1.79).

Women reported on all sources of their knowledge about family planning methods. In adjusted analyses, women who reported learning about methods from neighbors (51.4 %), doctors (46.5 %), nurses (35.6 %) or pharmacists (7.4 %) all had higher usage of modern family planning than women who did not report learning from these sources. There was no association between the use of modern family planning and learning about methods from media, including learning from books (1.9 %), magazines or newspapers (3.8 %), the internet (9.8 %), TV (9.5 %) or social media (2.8 %). Among women who had learned about family planning from their husbands (59.5 %), there was a 9 % reduction in the relative use of modern family planning compared to women who said they had not learned of family planning from their husbands, adjusting for having received counseling in the last 2 years, work status, lifetime births, wealth category, age and education level (aRR: 0.91, 95 % CI: 0.85–0.98). The examination of specific types in more detail shows that this reduction was primarily driven by a lower rate of IUD use.

4.2 Women's Concerns and Obstacles

Contraceptive trends differed by education, wealth status, awareness of methods and source of knowledge. We next examined whether women's contraceptive use differed by the feature of a contraceptive method they considered to be most important to see whether specific preferences or concerns led to the use of different specific types (Fig. 9.1). Concerns about health and side effects were commonly reported as the most important feature of a contraceptive method (43 %), followed by the effectiveness of the method (39 %). Very few women reported husband preference as the most important feature of contraception (<1 %). Women who considered effectiveness the most important feature had higher use of sterilization, IUD, and pills. Women who were concerned about the health effects of contraception had lower use of modern methods and higher use of withdrawal. Women who said they wanted a method that could be used without anyone knowing had the lowest rates of modern use and the highest rates of withdrawal. Nonuse was highest among women who prioritized wanting to be able to get pregnant again or who responded "don't know" regarding the most important feature, and these categories likely captured many women who wanted a pregnancy at the time of interview.

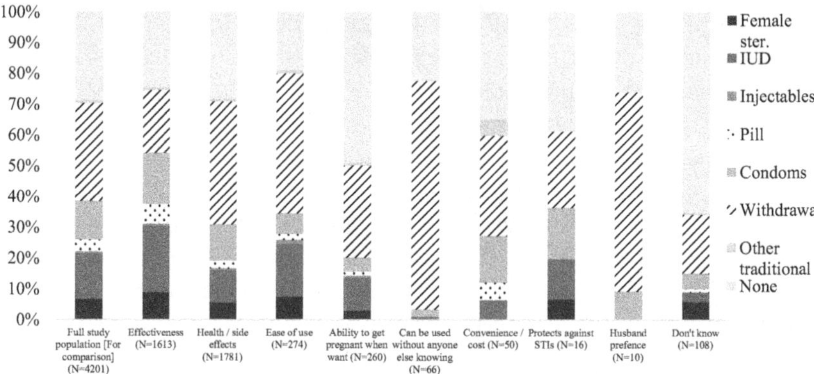

Fig. 9.1: Methods of contraception used, stratified by response to the question "In choosing a contraceptive method, what feature would be most important to you?". Proportions for each bar are age-standardized to the distribution of the study population.

The affordability of raising a child was indicated as a potential reason for using modern methods in the regression analyses that showed women in the lowest wealth quintile had higher use of modern contraception. While only 50 women stated cost or convenience as the most important feature of contraception (Fig. 9.1), these women had relatively higher use of condoms, pills, other traditional methods and no methods and lower use of sterilization and IUDs. When we stratified the sample by other reported concerns and obstacles, we found that 55 % of the study population reported that they would worry about the financial support for a child if they were to become pregnant in the next year or for the current pregnancy if they were currently pregnant. After adjusting for age, education, wealth index and lifetime births, women with financial worries were more likely to use contraception (aRR: 1.10, 95 % CI: 1.06–1.15), had higher use of IUD (aRR: 1.20, 95 % CI: 1.01–1.43), and had higher use of withdrawal (aRR: 1.14, 95 % CI: 1.03–1.26) than women who reported no financial worries. The results for financial concern and other reported concerns are displayed visually as age-standardized rates in Fig. 9.2.

Similarly, women who indicated hesitancy to become pregnant for various reasons had consistently higher use of contraception (Fig. 9.2). Women who looked forward to telling their husbands about their current or next pregnancy (50 % of the population) were less likely to use any contraception (aRR: 0.78, 95 % CI: 0.75–0.82), less likely to use permanent methods (aRR: 0.52, 95 % CI: 0.37–0.72), less likely to use IUDs (aRR: 0.80, 95 % CI: 0.68–0.95), and less likely to use withdrawal (aRR: 0.72, 95 % CI: 0.66–0.80). Women who looked forward to telling their parents about their current or next pregnancy (43 % of the population) were also less likely to use contraception (aRR: 0.75, 95 % CI: 0.72–0.79). Having health insurance (85 % of the population) had no impact on the use of modern contraception in the adjusted models.

In reports of obstacles to receiving family planning advice or treatment, having no one to look after children was reported as a main problem among 13 %, not wanting to go alone among 6 %, distance to the health facility among 5 %, obtaining the money needed for advice or treatment among 4 %, not having time because of work among 3 %, and obtaining permission to go to the doctor among 2 %. We investigated the obstacles endorsed by more than 5 % of women but did not see differing contraceptive prevalence for women who reported these problems (Fig. 9.2).

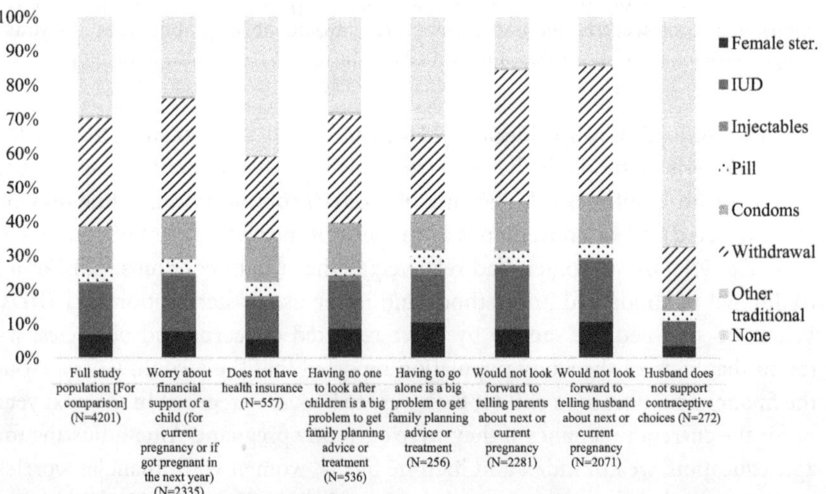

Fig. 9.2: Methods of contraception used among different segments of the study population based on responses to potential concerns and obstacles around family planning. The proportions for each bar are age-standardized to the distribution of the study population.

4.3 Women's Fertility Desires

The need for contraception in the population was high, with approximately half of the women in the study saying they wanted no more children and an additional 27 % wanting to wait at least 2 years until their next child (Tab. 9.3). Women most commonly stated that their lifetime desire for children would be 2 (26 %) or 3 (19 %) children, and a substantial number expressed the desire for zero children in their lifetime (15 %). There was no strong gender preference between wanting girls or boys. Wanting more children was associated with higher wealth, younger age, highest education and lowest education, fewer lifetime births, and husband support for the woman's contraceptive choices. The majority of women (68 %) stated that their husband wanted the same number of children as they did (Tab. 9.3).

Tab. 9.3: Frequency of responses to fertility desires and prevalence of unmet need for family planning

	N	**Percent**
Wants more children		
Wants another soon/within 2 years	456	10.8
Wants one later	1,150	27.2
Does not want any more	2,134	50.5
Reports cannot get pregnant	440	10.4
Missing	23	0.5
Refused	21	0.5
Total number of children desired over lifetime		
0	630	14.9
1	63	1.5
2	1,080	25.6
3	789	18.7
4	604	14.3
5+	109	2.6
Missing	22	0.5
Don't know	899	21.3
Refused	28	0.7
Wants at least one boy		
No/Does not care	2,987	70.7
Yes	1,215	28.8
Missing	22	0.5

(Continued)

Tab. 9.3: Continued

	N	Percent
Wants at least one girl		
No/Does not care	2,976	70.5
Yes	1,226	29.0
Missing	22	0.5
Husband desire for number of children		
Same number	2,855	67.6
More children	681	16.1
Fewer children	117	2.8
Don't know	535	12.7
	16	0.4
Refused	20	0.5
Unmet need for family planning		
Using modern contraception to limit	1,198	28.4
Using traditional contraception to limit	922	21.8
Using modern contraception to space	418	9.9
Using traditional contraception to space	450	10.7
Unmet need for limiting	227	5.4
Unmet need for spacing	196	4.6
No need	640	15.2
Infecund	134	3.2
Missing	39	0.9
Has unmet need		
No	3,762	89.1
Yes	423	10.0
Missing	39	0.9

Approximately 50 % of women used contraception for limiting births, and approximately 20 % used contraception for spacing births. Traditional methods were commonly used to meet family planning needs (Tab. 9.3). An unmet need for contraception was found among 10 % of women, half with an unmet need for limiting births and half with an unmet need for spacing births. Higher unmet need was associated with factors that were also associated with a lower desire for another child, including being in the oldest age group and already having 1–2 children (Tab. 9.4). Unmet need was also associated with the lowest education group and most notably with a lack of support from the husband in contraceptive choices, which was associated with a 5-fold higher risk of having unmet need (Tab. 9.4). The prevalence of contraceptive use by fertility desire group is displayed in Fig. 9.3 and shows the substantial proportion of women wanting to limit or space births who were using no methods or withdrawal for contraception. Different trends in choices of contraception were observed depending on whether the woman wanted to space or limit. Compared to those who wanted to limit births, those who wanted to space births had lower use of modern contraception (aRR: 0.85, 95 % CI: 0.77–0.94), lower use of IUD (aRR: 0.69, 95 % CI: 0.57–0.85), and higher use of condoms (aRR: 1.33, 95 % CI: 1.09–1.61).

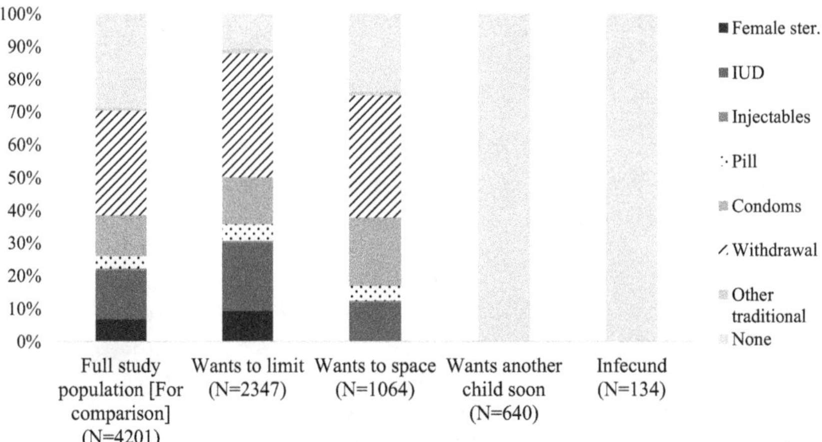

Fig. 9.3: Methods of contraception used, stratified by women's need for family planning. Proportions for each bar are age-standardized to the distribution of the study population.

Tab. 9.4: Predictors of unmet need for family planning

	RR (95 % CI)	p-value
Age category (ref: 35–39 years)		
16–19	1.66 (0.99, 2.80)	0.055
20–24	1.29 (0.88, 1.87)	0.192
25–29	1.02 (0.73, 1.41)	0.927
30–34	1.07 (0.8, 1.44)	0.635
40–44	1.74 (1.34, 2.25)	0.000
Education category (ref: Completed primary education)		
None/Primary incomplete	1.31 (1.05, 1.63)	0.016
Secondary school	0.85 (0.63, 1.15)	0.296
High school and higher	1.16 (0.88, 1.52)	0.291
Wealth quintile (ref: Poorest)		
Poorer	0.83 (0.60, 1.16)	0.277
Middle	0.82 (0.62, 1.09)	0.174
Richer	0.96 (0.74, 1.24)	0.745
Richest	1.03 (0.77, 1.39)	0.829
Number of lifetime births (ref: 0)		
1	1.59 (1.17, 2.16)	0.003
2	1.26 (0.93, 1.72)	0.141
3	1.07 (0.76, 1.51)	0.698
4	0.90 (0.59, 1.37)	0.631
5+	0.82 (0.53, 1.28)	0.386
Husband supports woman's contraceptive choices (ref: Yes)		
No	4.99 (4.12, 6.05)	0.000

4.4 Husbands' Desires and Support

Next, we consider the role of the husband's fertility desires and support in women's contraceptive choices in more depth. Women reported that their husbands were employed (98 %) and literate (99 %). Husbands were commonly 1–5 years older than the women (52 %). Among 20 % of women, the husband was 6–10 years older, and among 7 % of women, the husband was >10 years older. A kin marriage was reported among 10 % of women. Most women (93 %) reported that their husband was supportive of their contraceptive choices, and among women using contraception, 97 % reported that their husband knew they were using contraception. There were no associations found in chi-square tests between husband support and age at first cohabitation, age difference between the woman and the husband, or kin marriage. Reports of husband support were associated with women's age category (chi-square p = 0.001), with women in the 16–19 age range reporting lower husband support (80 %) than women in all other age ranges (>90 %). Reports of husband support were highest among women who said their husband desired the same number of children they did (96 %) and lowest among women who said they did not know whether their husband desired the same number of children (81 %; chi-square p < 0.001).

Husbands' desire for children relative to the women's desire was not a strong predictor of contraceptive choice, although women who said that they did not know whether their husband wanted the same number of children reported a lower use of contraception than women whose husbands wanted the same number (aRR: 0.87, 95 % CI: 0.82–0.93). On the other hand, lack of husband support in women's contraceptive choices was highly correlated with lower contraceptive use (Fig. 9.2). Women who reported support in contraceptive choices from their husband had higher use of modern contraception (aRR: 1.96, 95 % CI: 1.50–2.56), IUDs (aRR: 1.92, 95 % CI: 1.21–3.04), condoms (aRR: 2.98, 95 % CI: 1.60–5.53), and withdrawal (aRR: 1.99, 95 % CI: 1.48–2.69) than women who did not report husband support.

When examining whether contraceptive choices based on women's fertility desire differed by either the husband's support or the husband's fertility desire, there was no clear association between contraceptive use and the interaction between husbands' fertility desire and women's fertility desire. However, the interaction between women's fertility desire and husbands' support of contraceptive choices showed a clear impact on contraceptive use (Fig. 9.4). Among women who wanted to limit births, lack of husband support led to a 42 % reduction in use of any contraception (aRR: 0.58, 95 % CI: 0.49–0.69), as well as a reduction in relative use of modern contraception (aRR: 0.59, 95 % CI: 0.44–0.79), condoms (aRR: 0.35, 95 % CI: 0.15–0.83), and withdrawal (aRR: 0.56, 95 % CI: 0.39–0.80). There was a slight reduction in the use of female sterilization, IUD and pills, but these differences were not statistically significant. Among women who wanted to space their next birth, those who reported lack of support from their husband had lower use of contraception overall (aRR: 0.38, 95 % CI: 0.27–0.53), lower use of modern contraception (aRR: 0.35, 95 % CI: 0.49–0.90), lower use of IUD (aRR: 0.38, 95 % CI: 0.14–0.99), lower use of condoms (aRR: 0.29, 95 % CI: 0.12–0.69), and lower use of withdrawal (aRR: 0.41, 95 % CI: 0.24–0.68), as well as slightly lower use of pills, which was not statistically significant. Figure 9.4 displays age-standardized comparisons of the prevalence of use of each of the contraceptive types for these groups of women: wants to limit births and has husband's support, wants to limit births and lacks husband's support, wants to space next birth and has husband's support, wants to space next birth and lacks husband's support.

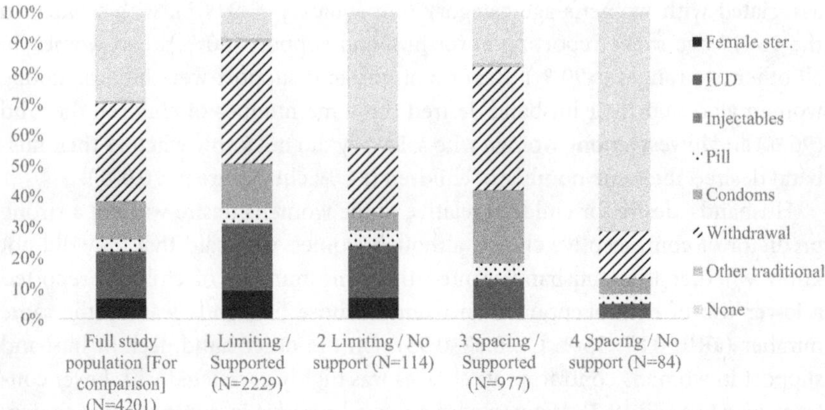

Fig. 9.4: Methods of contraception used among women wanting to limit or space births, stratified by women's need for family planning and husband's support in choice of contraception. Proportions for each bar are age-standardized to the distribution of the study population.

5 Discussion

5.1 Themes

The study population was similar to that observed in national data from Turkey regarding the prevalence of use of contraceptive types and high awareness of contraceptive methods overall (DHS, 2014). Several important themes around factors that impact contraceptive choices emerged from these data, which may have significance for understanding and improving the contraceptive choices of women throughout Turkey, particularly women living in poorer urban neighborhoods.

We observed that trends in contraceptive choices correlated with women's fertility desires and hesitancy toward pregnancy; for example, women who wanted to limit pregnancy were more likely to use long-acting methods than those who wanted to space pregnancies. However, there were still a substantial number of women who wanted to limit or space their next pregnancy and who did not use contraception. Additionally, women who did use family planning relied heavily upon an unreliable method, withdrawal, as their primary means for contraception. Given the relatively high reports of unwanted pregnancies in Turkey (DHS, 2014), this implies that many women need more effective methods. Even women who prioritized effectiveness as the most important feature of a contraceptive method used withdrawal, with a prevalence of 20 %. Use of withdrawal was particularly high for women who prioritized contraception that featured ease of use, lack of side effects, or the possibility of use without anyone else knowing, suggesting that these issues should be addressed in family planning counseling.

Other problems in accessing family planning were reported with low frequency or did not lead to any substantial impact on contraceptive prevalence, for example, for women who reported childcare or not wanting to go alone as a problem in accessing family planning advice or treatment. A substantial portion of the population had financial worries about supporting a child, yet the cost of a contraceptive method itself did not appear to be a barrier in accessing contraception. Lack of health insurance was not very impactful on contraceptive rates, very few women prioritized the cost of a method in choosing contraception, and very few identified costs as a major problem in accessing family planning. Lower wealth and financial concerns around raising a child, however, resulted in lower fertility desire and higher use of all types of contraception.

The results also revealed an opportunity for improvement in education, counseling and awareness of methods. Women with higher education had greater awareness of alternative contraceptive methods, and those with greater awareness of different types of methods were more likely to be currently using modern contraception even after controlling for education level, age, wealth, number of lifetime births, and recent contraceptive counseling. These results are consistent with the idea that awareness and education are associated with better power to choose contraceptive methods that fit with a woman's preferences, as previous research suggests that this leads to improved continuity of contraceptive use (Marshall et al., 2015). Despite the already high level of awareness of contraception in Turkey, improvement in education on the availability of different types of methods could help women achieve their family planning goals.

We also observed that there was the opportunity for healthcare professionals to reach more women for counseling and education on family planning methods during their visits to healthcare facilities. As previous research indicates the possibility for pharmacists to play a stronger role in family planning counseling for women in Turkey (Özaydın et al., 2020), we also observed that receiving counseling from healthcare providers was associated with higher modern method use and lower traditional method use. This trend may be due to the lack of demand for counseling among women who are not interested in modern contraception or women who miss out on counseling during contacts with the healthcare system, leading to lower awareness of available methods and their risks and benefits when choosing contraception. The results also demonstrated higher modern contraception use among women whose source of knowledge about family planning came from doctors, nurses or pharmacists. We also note that there was elevated use of modern contraception among women who had learned about family planning from neighbors, indicating that in addition to healthcare professionals, social networks can be a valuable source for improving awareness of different methods.

Lastly, the results regarding the role of the husband showed that most women felt supported by their husbands in their choice of contraception, and very few identified their husbands' preference as the most important feature of contraception. However, for women who did not feel supported by their husbands regarding contraception choices, husband support was a very significant obstacle. Not having their husband's support was one of the strongest predictors of nonuse of contraception among all of the obstacles and concerns evaluated. Lack of husband support was especially impactful for women who wanted to space childbirth and for methods that men control (condoms, withdrawal), which are very prevalent in Turkey. Notably, learning about family planning from a husband or partner was reported frequently and was the only family planning information source associated with lower use of modern methods. The results suggest vulnerability among women in the youngest age range (<20 years old), among whom 20 % reported a lack of support from their husbands, and emphasize the importance of men's involvement and support in family planning.

5.2 Limitations and Implications

This study was limited given that the geographic coverage of the study population included only two districts in Istanbul, but given the similarities in contraceptive use to the population of Turkey, we believe inferences can be made that can inform and support women's contraceptive decision making in poor urban areas throughout Istanbul and Turkey. The cross-sectional nature of the survey also implies that the data reported here demonstrate associations that cannot be interpreted as strictly causal. We also have limited ability to identify additional obstacles or important factors influencing the choice of contraception that were not specifically addressed in the survey, given the close-ended nature of the questions.

The results demonstrate that there is opportunity for improvement in women's awareness and ability to choose more effective contraceptive methods in Turkey. Specifically, we highlight the importance of the husband's support of contraceptive choices, improving education about the available types of methods, and providing opportunities for family planning counseling for reproductive-aged women when they have contact with the healthcare system. These factors should be considered to inform health policies for reproductive-aged women in Turkey.

References

Ayaz, S., & Efe, S. Y. (2009). Family planning attitudes of women and affecting factors. *Journal of the Turkish German Gynecological Association, 10*(3), 137–141.

Bradley, S. E. K., Croft, T. N., Fishel, J. D., & Westoff, C. F. (2012). Revising unmet need for family planning. *DHS Analytical Studies,* No. 25. Calverton, ICF International.

Çalıkoğlu, E. O., Yerli, E. B., Kavuncuoğlu, D., Yılmaz, S., Koşan, Z., & Aras A. (2018). Use of family planning methods and influencing factors among women in Erzurum. *Medical Science Monitor, 24,* 5027–5034.

DHS Turkey. Hacettepe University Institute of Population Studies. (2014). 2013 Turkey Demographic and Health Survey. *Hacettepe University Institute of Population Studies,* T.R. Ministry of Development and TÜBITAK, Ankara, Turkey.

Foster, A. M., & Doci, F. (2017). Factors influencing women's contraceptive decision-making in Albania: Florida Doci. *European Journal of Public Health, 27*(suppl_3), 162–163.

Marshall, C., Guendelman, S., Mauldon, J., & Nuru-Jeter, A. (2015). Women's contraceptive decision making: How well do women's preferences for certain contraceptive attributes align with the methods they use? *Contraception, 92*(4), 383–384.

Özaydın, A. N., Bozdoğan, B., Kıcı N., & Özaydın, F. N. (2020). The availability of contraceptive methods in Turkish pharmacies and the status of pharmacies and pharmacists as providers of contraception. *The European Journal of Contraception & Reproductive Health Care, 25*(6), 427–433.

Özdemir, R., Çevik, C., & Çiçeklioğlu, M. (2019). Unmet needs for family planning among married women aged 15–49 years living in two settlements with different socioeconomic and cultural characteristics: A cross-sectional study from Karabuk Province in Turkey. *Rural and Remote Health, 19*(3), 5125.

United Nations, Department of Economic and Social Affairs, Population Division. (2015). *Trends in contraceptive use worldwide 2015* (ST/ESA/SER.A/349).

Yılmazel, G., Çetinkaya, F., Nacar, M., & Baykan, Z. (2019). Which men have better attitudes and participation to family planning services? A study in primary care settings from Northern Turkey. *Nigerian Journal of Clinical Practice, 22*(8), 1055–1062.

Yücel, U., Çiçeklioğlu, M., Öcek, Z. A., & Varol, Z. S. (2020). Access to primary health care family planning services and contraceptive use in disadvantaged women: A qualitative study. *The European Journal of Contraception & Reproductive Health Care, 25*(5), 327–333.

www.ingramcontent.com/pod-product-compliance
Lightning Source LLC
Chambersburg PA
CBHW031541260326
41914CB00002B/208

* 9 7 8 3 6 3 1 8 4 8 9 0 6 *